Thriving THROUGH Infertility

Contributing Authors

Lindsay Alvut, Monica Bivas, Nicole Buratti, Dr. Celeste Brabec,
Michelle Byrd, Dr. L. April Gago, Amy Green, Lyle Harvey,
Dr. Kristin Lasseter, Michelle Oravitz, Cathie Quillet,
Dr. Dan Schaefer, Lisa Schuman, Dr. Mark Trolice
and Dr. Melissa Wenrich

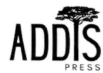

© 2021 Addis Press
The Quillet Institute
www.thequilletinstitute.com
ISBN 979-8-573-05672-2

This book is dedicated to

Every Fertility Warrior

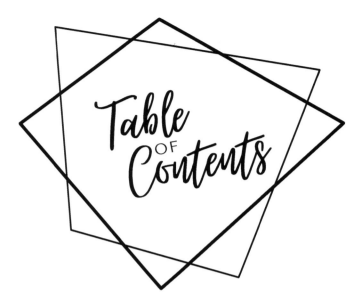

Table OF Contents

Introduction

By Cathie Quillet

"I'm so sorry, Mrs. Quillet. You are infertile."

I remember those words like it was yesterday.

In that moment, my world fell off its axis. Grief intersected with my life even though the only thing that I had lost were the plans and expectations that I had for my life.

In that moment, all of my peers became better women than me, even though the only place where that reality existed was in my perception of my own worth.

In that moment, I surrendered our biological legacy, becoming an utter disappointment to both sides of our family, even though I was the only one disappointed me in.

In that moment, I became part of a club, one that is the most beautiful of clubs even though no one wants to claim membership in it.

In that moment and through the end of our fertility journey, I felt completely lost. Broken. In shambles.

Have you been there?

Are you there now?

It is in these fragile moments that we fasten our seatbelt and put our life on cruise control with the expectation of mere survival. We surrender the idea of living our best lives, put our heads down, wipe our tears, and just try to get through it.

Thriving is now something fertile people do.

Thriving is something that you will do again, but only once you have your baby.

But what if I told you that thriving is possible NOW, in the midst of angst, anxiety and apathy.

Assembled in this book is the heart work of professionals in the field of fertility. Together, our motivation is to help you thrive. Not when baby comes or when you finally have a viable pregnancy, but right now, right in the middle of infertility.

Thriving through infertility does not minimize the reality that infertility is a trauma; rather, it says that I am fighting for myself as much as I am fighting for a baby.

We want you to be able to look back on your season of infertility and say "I lived well. I thrived."

When the Struggle is Real Right Out of the Gate

By Lindsay Alvut

Mental health struggles can pop up at any stage of the family planning journey. For folks who already have a long history of anxiety, depression, etc., the stress of encountering complications with growing a family can cause great distress. Based on my personal experience and the experiences I have heard from many of my clients, it can be surprising how strong the emotional struggle can become early on. For some, even before an official diagnosis of infertility. Sometimes there may be key events that occur which lead people to seek professional mental health support (formal infertility diagnosis, transfer of care from OB/GYN to infertility doctor, the start of IUI/IVF, pregnancy loss, etc). However, I am here to encourage folks to reach out for support as soon as it makes sense for you.

I'm a fairly healthy person, but I have a history of endometriosis and fibroids. Because of this, I didn't want to wait too long to start trying to get pregnant in case we encountered fertility challenges that I'd read could be associated with those conditions. I planned when we could start trying to have a baby and diligently waited until the month came where I knew I wouldn't mess up my graduation plans if I went into labor early. I knew exactly when we were in the clear to get things going. I was focused.

I prepared myself to be pleasantly surprised that we would get pregnant after our first month of trying it stung a little bit when we didn't. Each month that went by felt exponentially worse and my preexisting anxiety jumped right into high gear. Was I being punished for choosing to get my degree when I should have used that time to get pregnant? Was it too late?

During these initial months of trying to become pregnant, I became fluent in the language of infertility (TTC, TWW, IUI, IVF, etc. If you're reading this, you are probably already well aware). Not because I was diagnosed with infertility yet, but because my anxiety and perfectionism made me overly ambitious and cautiously on guard that something would go terribly wrong straight out of the gate. I started buying cheap pregnancy strips online in bulk and I would test numerous times a day. I googled and researched and armed myself not only with useful information but also with worst-case scenarios, loss, and stories of trauma. Looking back, I can clearly identify that these were compulsive ways of managing anxiety and obsessive thoughts about getting pregnant.

Then after several months of negative pregnancy tests, I used a digital pregnancy test one morning. This was a very rare occurrence because, like I said, I'd been using the very cheap pregnancy strips that I bought in bulk. By gosh, it read, "pregnant"! My stomach fell through my knees! Right there plain as day, not up for interpretation. Pregnant. I'd fallen through several rabbit holes watching cute pregnancy announcements on YouTube in preparation for this very moment (the awful, terrible, horrible, deplorable, dreaded two-week wait gives you the opportunity to google way too much). I briefly considered orchestrating a cute announcement for my husband later that day, but I just couldn't wait. I ran up the stairs and approached his side of the bed and showed him the positive test. I remember my due date was 11/11 which I thought was absolutely, wonderfully perfect.

We ended up losing the pregnancy.

The International Committee Monitoring Assisted Reproductive Technologies (ICMART) defines infertility as a disease that is characterized by the inability to establish a clinical pregnancy after 12 months of regular unprotected intercourse, or due to an impairment of a person's ability to reproduce as an individual or with their partner. They go on to define that fertility interventions may be started under one year based on medical, sexual and reproductive history, age, physical findings, and diagnostic testing. (1)

These guidelines are helpful for physicians to identify treatment options for the physical impact of infertility. However, the mental health impact doesn't necessarily follow suit with these timelines, especially if you have preexisting conditions. Based on personal and clinical experience, I understand that plenty of folks begin struggling with the impact of trying for a baby well before a clinical diagnosis of infertility is established. In my case, I felt validated enough by my early pregnancy loss, endometriosis, and fibroids to advocate for more aggressive physical treatment options. I never considered, however, that maybe I could have advocated for some emotional support as well.

At this time, I established care with an infertility doctor. I was way too impatient to allow this nonsense to go on for another six months before asking for help. I'd love to share with you the details about timelines and treatments, but much of it is a blur. In retrospect, I believe my spotty memory has been a trauma response and a natural act of self-protection.

(1) International Committee Monitoring Assisted Reproductive Technologies (ICMART) (2012-2019). Glossary: The International Glossery on Infertility and Fertility Care. icmartivf.org.

I was prescribed different medications, first oral, and then injectable. My first IUI was unsuccessful. I'd blown through those cheap pregnancy strips by the dozens. I'd constantly dig them out of the garbage to study them for faint lines. I was compulsive. My brain understood that testing over and over throughout the day would not change the results, but the compulsion was deeply rooted in a long history of anxiety, and the distress around becoming and staying pregnant exacerbated my anxious thoughts and compulsive actions. The details are a blur, but I miscarried two more times. All three of the pregnancies were lost very early on, which was heartbreaking and confusing.

The worst part was that I felt unjustified in my pain and suffering. I was watching myself flail, and I started to self-loathe. I am very introverted at baseline, and I began isolating myself even more. I snapped at the people I loved. I didn't feel like myself anymore. But more than anything, I hated myself for feeling that much pain in the first place. I'd earned my degree as a therapist, which made me think, "I have the skills to navigate this, what is wrong with me?" This self-talk leads to feelings of being a fraud professionally, as well.

But the thing is, my mental health was NOT well. My anxiety and obsessive-compulsive tendencies were thriving. I was going through numerous pregnancy test strips per day and compulsively googling. My thoughts felt like a looped tape at top volume. Due to the timelines being so early, I shamed myself. I compared myself to other women I'd read about who were stronger and more resilient, communicating messages of hope after grueling treatments, IVF, surrogacy, loss, and adoption. What was wrong with me? I hadn't been struggling with this for long enough to justify my emotional state. If this were the suffering olympics, my emotions were earning a gold but my physical journey hadn't even earned me placement as an honorable mention. I felt such shame.

I believe that a vast number of infertility sufferers feel they cannot validate the significant feelings of trauma, loss, and grief early on in the infertility process because they compare themselves to others who have suffered for longer or have experienced 'worse'. If this can be challenged early on, I feel that individuals and couples will be more adept at recognizing pain for what it is with less judgment. Then they can allow themselves the much-needed grace to learn tools to self-soothe and cope in ways that are kinder toward themselves.

The thing about infertility is that you don't know how long it will last. Only upon looking back and reflecting on your journey can you make sense of your experience. You don't need to wait until your journey is over to do this reflection. Simply look back at your experiences thus far and ask yourself if you've shown signs of emotional struggle. If you have, you may benefit from additional support, wherever you are in the process of family building. Jaffe & Diamond (2011) explain that "it is important for people to be with others who truly understand and can identify with their pain and trauma".2 Working with a therapist with specialized training and experience in the nuance of infertility is important.

My final IUI was successful. The night before I got the positive pregnancy test, I remember actively pushing away fear-based self-talk that told me not to exercise because it would somehow cause me to lose the potential pregnancy. Instead, I went into my partially finished basement, put on some noise-canceling headphones, and danced in the dark by the glow of the TV. This was pretty out of my character, but it felt like a way to honor the struggle I had been through. I allowed myself to flail around to some really loud techno-pop and dance away the negativity. I now remember that memory as being one of my first bonding moments with my daughter. Who, you will be glad to know, has her mommy's terrible dance moves.

2 https://www.icmartivf.org/glossary/i-m/ Jaffe, J., & Diamond M. O.2011. Reproductive Trauma: Psychotherapy With Infertility and Pregnancy Loss Clients. Washington, DC: American Psychological Association. pg 63.

I faced a lot of emotional challenges while building my family. My recurrent losses impacted my experience and enjoyment of my 4th and 5th pregnancies. I struggled with postpartum anxiety after having my first child. While I didn't struggle to become and stay pregnant with my second born, I carried residual emotional baggage with me through the pregnancy anyway.

Both of my deliveries resulted in admissions to intensive care units at the hospital. I became very ill and ended up in the ICU after my first delivery. Then, my second baby was born with a hole in their lung which resulted in an emergency transfer to a hospital with NICU facilities. I was separated from both of my babies after their births and I didn't have typical bonding experiences with either of them. These experiences impacted my opportunity to emotionally bond with my babies in a traditional way, and in one of the cases, the separation had a long-term impact on my milk supply which resulted in plenty of additional emotional struggles for myself and my partner.

For myself (and for many) the emotional challenges don't fizzle away with a positive pregnancy test. Experiences can compound on top of one another if they are not dealt with in a helpful way.

I've learned that building your family can be beautiful. It can also be painful, grief-ridden, and filled with jealousy. It can be filled with unexpected outcomes. It can leave you feeling guilty when you have something to celebrate while you are in the midst of a friend or family member who is experiencing loss. Building a family can be massively and emotionally complicated. In other ways, it can also be simple and joyful.

Through my extensive work with this population, it is repeatedly reinforced that are no two family-building journeys that look the same. I believe that establishing a relationship with a therapist who specializes in

Infertility and Perinatal Mental Health is the best way to feel truly supported with your specific experience and needs along the way.

While my experience may look very different from yours, I have cobbled together years of personal and professional experience. This work is my passion, and I truly believe it is possible to have a fruitful life and to thrive through infertility (and beyond!).

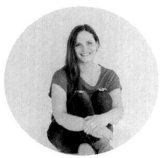

lindsay Alvut
Licensed Mental Health Counselor
www.lindsayalvut.com

Lindsay Alvut (she/hers) is a Licensed Mental Health Counselor who operates her private practice, Lindsay Alvut Mental Health Counseling, PLLC in the greater Rochester, NY area. She specializes in Infertility and Perinatal Mental Health and offers telehealth to folks throughout the state of New York.

When she isn't working she loves spending time with her family, drinking coffee, crafting, reading, and listening to true crime podcasts. To work with Lindsay please visit https://www.lindsayalvut.com/contact and fill out a contact form.

IVF is a Journey, Not a Destination

By Monica Bivas

In vitro fertilization (IVF) has been a blessing in my life. However, it is also a roller-coaster ride of emotions. With constant changes in the treatment itself, there is a lot of information to absorb. IVF treatments today are not the same as they were five years, three years, or even one year ago. Every day there is more and more research on fertility treatments to help those suffering from fertility issues, allowing not only the greater possibility of getting pregnant but having a healthy pregnancy and a healthy baby.

With IVF comes many emotions, including a sense of being overwhelmed and confused. My first three cycles were extremely stressful and difficult. My third IVF cycle ended with the stillbirth of my beautiful baby girl at thirty-nine weeks, just three days before her expected due date. I did my fourth cycle almost immediately after my stillbirth, and even after having a big fat positive (BFP), I miscarried at seven weeks.

I realized that, in order to handle another round of IVF, I would have to take control of the situation based on what I'd lived through in previous cycles. To me, this meant knowing and accepting my medical situation. I have double tube blockage caused by endometriosis. Even after a laparoscopy, they remain blocked. I also have to know and accept my menstrual cycles, my body, my feelings, and my relationship with my partner.

My last cycle resulted in the birth of my second daughter, Maya, and my first IVF cycle was also successful, culminating with the birth of my daughter, Eliyah.

Based on my own experience through IVF is why I decided to be a collaborator in this book, and provide information that can help others walking this same path and find the best tools that could bring them to a positive outcome, which is not only to get a positive pregnancy test but a live baby in their arms.

Before you start, I have some general suggestions for maintaining a positive attitude and managing your treatment: don't compare yourself to others. Every single woman going through IVF is different, and each cycle is different. What is normal for you might not be for other women. In IVF, there is no right or wrong.

Similarly, every reproductive endocrinologist (RE) and clinic is different. Your diagnosis and IVF experience depends on the clinic you choose. Your diagnosis will differ depending on the specialty of the RE, the cause of your infertility, and the number of times you have gone through IVF. However, as long as you are comfortable and receive kind, understanding care, all can go smoothly.

Remember, it is very important that you check on the success rate of the clinic. Not on the positive tests, but on the live birth pregnancies they have. That is what it counts regarding this specific subject, and then you can go from there.

Prepare, but don't make plans based on an anticipated outcome. IVF has many variables. The timing of each step can change, and the outcome is not certain until the very end. What you can do, though, is prepare for the experience.

Get your information directly from the source. If you have any type of question, don't rely on Google or other medical personnel. You will receive conflicting information that will only confuse and overwhelm you. Your RE and his or her team should be able to answer any questions you have, relieve your doubts, and give you the advice you need. Never let information from insensitive or unverified sources confuse you. This will only bring you unnecessary stress. Remember that you also have a say in your cycle.

IVF treatment options are continually evolving with new research and the discovery of new medicines. This is wonderful because it increases the possibility of a big fat positive (BFP) result and a healthy, full-term pregnancy. It can also affect how you interact with REs and clinics in terms of your finances.

Learn the basics of IVF treatment. In vitro fertilization (IVF) places a woman's egg and a man's sperm in a laboratory dish for the purpose of creating a viable embryo. The fertilized eggs become embryos, and then several, based on how many are viable, are placed in the woman's uterus, where they hopefully will implant.

Every cycle is different, but most follow a basic system. To be prepared for your specific situation, you must understand how the cycle works.

The cycle has steps such as pre-cycle, stimulation, egg retrieval, and sperm collection, fertilization & growth, and embryo transfer and results. All of these together bring our cycle to an outcome, which can be a positive one. It also can develop into a full-term pregnancy or sometimes in miscarriage. If the outcome is a miscarriage, then the best thing for you to do is to take time to grieve and heal. Then decide if you should go through another cycle of IVF.

Not knowing what to expect can be stressful and make the treatment more difficult. The outcome of an IVF cycle is always unknown, so don't focus on the "what ifs" or your worries about it. Instead, I suggest you focus on the treatment positively and calmly. How? Make your best effort to understand the treatment itself, your diagnosis, and all the possible outcomes before you even start. By doing this, you demystify your treatment and are more mentally prepared for any possible outcome.

IVF treatments generally follow a basic timeline, but they can still be unpredictable. Unexpected changes can create stress and uncertainty when they force you to alter your schedule. I recommend adopting a flexible mindset, so you are less bothered by unexpected changes. Art therapy, meditation, acupuncture, and light yoga were some of the things I started to practice to help me become calmer.

Waiting is also something you must be prepared for. IVF involves a lot of time spent waiting, which can be very time-consuming. If you work, my suggestion is to give notice to your manager about your IVF treatment. If you don't work and are a housewife, organize your schedule so that you have flexibility.

Think about IVF as a Journey, not a destination. IVF cycles are not quick treatments. There can be many months between finding out if this is your only treatment option and the conclusion of an IVF cycle. In some complicated cases, treatment can take years.

I am not saying this to scare you. I just want to prepare you in case your treatment takes longer than you expected. This is why I call it a journey. You can find more information about the success rates of IVF cycles at the Society for Assisted Reproductive Technology's website (www.sart.org).

Find a Network and Support Groups

The fertility community is incredible. There are so many options to get the right support. One of the blessings IVF brought into my life was my decision to become a Mindset & Holistic Fertility Coach. I have met the most wonderful people in this community, where we have support while knowing we are not alone. That can play a huge role in the outcome of our cycle, so it is important to know that there is nothing to be embarrassed about, you did nothing wrong, and you are not the only one walking this path.

IVF treatment may be the hardest thing you've ever done, but know you're not alone. Going through IVF treatment is simultaneously the easiest and hardest thing you'll ever do. Deciding to go through treatment can be an easy choice, but dealing with the emotions that emerge and keeping track of all the information can be daunting.

An IVF journey, no matter what the result; negative, positive, or canceled cycles, takes strength, courage, and somehow teaches us to be disciplined. It teaches us lessons of patience, love, and understanding. One of the most important things is not to forget where you were before you started this journey. Yes, the ultimate goal is to have your baby in your arms, but make sure you nourish yourself. If you are in a good place or try your best to build the best environment for yourself while you walk this journey, you are moving forward towards a positive outcome.

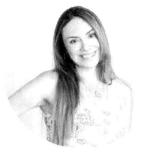

Monica Bivas
Mindset & Holistic Fertility Coach
www.monicabivas.com

Monica Bivas is a Mindset & Holistic Fertility Coach, speaker, writer of the Book The IVF Planner and founder of The IVF Journey, an online community for women and couples to find support, hope, and connection with other individuals contemplating or experiencing In Vitro Fertilization.

Monica is a Certified Fertility coach from the Wholesome Fertility Program and specializes in Mindset and Emotional Support for Individuals and couples Trying to Conceive Via ART, like IVF or IUI, as well as emotional support in Pregnancy and Infant loss.

Monica was a regular contributor to the Huffington Post, Thrive Global and has been a host in multiple Fertility Podcasts, where she talks about her own journey, and planning for and managing IVF treatments, as well on support on TTC naturally.

Her book, The IVF Planner, is a journal and guide for women undergoing fertility treatment and has another book forthcoming about her life-changing experience with IVF treatment and her Stillbirth and loss experience at 39 weeks of her baby daughter Isabelle as well as her following miscarriage at 7 weeks after trying again IVF.

Diagnosed with Infertility? Summarizing it All While Keeping it Human

By Dr. Celeste Brabec

If there is one thing that we know well, it is that an infertility diagnosis can be shocking and extremely overwhelming. Many ask themselves, "why me?" or, "what now?" You are not alone. Let's walk through this new world of infertility that you are about to experience, all while keeping it realistic.

Step 1: Relax in the Facts

The good news is, if you want to get pregnant and start a family, the odds are greatly in your favor that you will achieve your goal. So before taking one step forward, take a deep sigh of relief in that fact. When you start to feel tense, fall back on that thought as a soft place to land at the end of the day. We all need and deserve that.

Step 2: Take Control and Do Your Research

Control is in your grasp. Seize the opportunity of that control. Keeping a sense of control over your choices is important to feel at peace.

While letting fate or time or someone else set your destination takes the pressure off of your back, doing so relinquishes your control and contributes to stress. It is like getting into a rideshare and telling the driver to take you wherever they are already going, and then getting mad that you didn't end up where you wanted to go. Instead, allow yourself to take a risk in admitting that you want a baby. Admitting it takes guts because there is a risk of failure. Let's say your goal is to have a baby. Set your "destination" to that goal, and research the different routes to get there, each with its time estimate to reach the destination, like any map app on your phone.

Options for infertility treatment will include:

1) Do nothing.
Doing nothing is always an option. Keep in mind some general numbers. In fully fertile couples, the odds of getting pregnant in one month are not 100%, even if eggs, sperm, tubes, and uterus are normal. In fully fertile couples, pregnancy rates are estimated to be approximately 15% when the female age is under 35, approximately 9% per month with the female age 35-39, and under 1% with the female age 40+. Yes, those stats apply to the fully fertile population. The odds of getting pregnant in one month by doing nothing if you have infertility are under 2%. Not zero, but not great. And, if you choose to do nothing, make it a willful choice, not a surrendering, "Woe is me. It just wasn't meant to be."

2) Oral medication with intrauterine insemination (OI-IUI).
This option requires at least one normal fallopian tube and a not too bad semen analysis. Pregnancy rates are in the range of 5-15% per cycle, depending on your age and diagnosis.

3) In Vitro Fertilization (IVF)
This option is available even if both fallopian tubes are blocked, tied,

non-functional, or surgically absent. IVF is also an option for those with moderate to severe endometriosis and with severe compromise in semen analysis. It requires at least one functional ovary, at least a few sperm, and a uterus. Variations under the umbrella of IVF may have success rates of over 70% in one cycle, but success is very dependent on the female's age and diagnosis. I sometimes refer to IVF as flying instead of driving to your destination. If your ovaries can respond well to fertility medication, then doing one IVF cycle may be thought of as the equivalent of doing 10+ cycles of oral medication with IUI. IVF can be a better choice than OI-IUI if time is of the essence. IVF has a lower multiple-rate than oral medication with IUI. The downside? IVF is costly. But so are tears and time. Be sure to weigh your options according to your needs and desires.

4) Third-Party (Donor Egg, Donor Sperm, Host Uterus)
Third-party reproduction is an option when these are absent or compromised in function. Sometimes, we use all three treatments at the same time. While third party reproduction is not first on the list for most individuals, it is an option that significantly raises the chances of having a family.

5) Adoption
Adoption is another option for your consideration. Each choice has advantages and disadvantages. Keep in mind that adoption can be more costly than all of the other options, including IVF. Adoption does not have a 100% success and may entail scrutiny of your suitability to become a parent, which is hard for some.

Step 3: Expect the Unexpected

There is not a 100% chance of success, zero risk, or zero cost. Things can and will go wrong. There will be detours along the way. Most likely, you've already faced some of these detours. Maybe your heart is set on delivering a baby during a specific time of year. Or maybe that you must have your egg retrieval on Tuesday because other obligations make Wednesday more challenging. Or you feel you simply must be pregnant before the holidays. Fertility does not always align with your schedule and desires, but it will be okay. Find ways to laugh, accept the detours, and move forward. Seek ways to thrive in the midst of infertility despite all that may go awry during this season of life.

Step 4: Set Limits

How much time do you have? How much money? How much emotional tenacity? Like setting your budget for your wedding, house, car, or vacation, think about the resources you feel comfortable allotting to the goal of having a baby to help you choose the path best for you. You know you better than any doctor, friend, or book knows you.

Infertility and fertility treatment can be all-consuming. Should we go on vacation? I might be ovulating that week! Should we buy a house? We need to wait to see how many bedrooms we need! Of course, you will need to talk about and think about fertility.

When you must worry and talk and cry and discuss fertility, set a time frame. I suggest one hour a day. Give yourself one hour a day to think about, talk about, and cry about fertility. Wall off this time like your body walls off an abscess to prevent infection from taking over the entire body. The other 23 hours, focus on something else. Otherwise, infertility will fester, grow, and consume your life. Do not let it.

Step 5: Have Fun!

Wear your best lingerie just for yourself. Spray on some perfume. Glide on your favorite lip balm. Giggle. Cuddle. Be sweet and kind to each other. Get some fresh air, exercise, and keep your spiritual life strong. Keep family, friends, and acquaintances in your social arena (you can decide whether or not you share your infertility journey with them). Keep a hobby. Let the science of medications, schedules, and treatments go at times, and just be together for the sheer pleasure of it, without the goal of pregnancy looming over every interaction.

No matter how things turn out, picture yourself at age eighty. Do you have a family? Are you child free? Even if it didn't turn out as you desired, do you feel good about the information you got and the choices you made? If so, I predict you will find happiness, contentment, and peace.

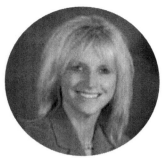

Dr. Celeste Brabec
Reproductive Endocrinologist
www.rrc.com

Celeste Brabec, M.D. is a Fellowship-Trained, Board Certified Reproductive Endocrinologist. She completed medical training at the University of Texas Health Science Center at Houston, Residency at Creighton University in Omaha and her Fellowship in Infertility at Harvard in 1997. She joined RRC in 1999 and now serves as Medical Director. Dr. Brabec's focus is the face-to-face care of couples and individuals with fertility issues. Dr. Brabec is a member of the prestigious Alpha Omega Alpha Medical Honor Society. She has been voted "Super Doctor in Infertility" by her local peers, as well as nationally designated one of "America's Top Obstetricians and Gynecologists", for many years running, and has been listed on "Who's Who in the 21st Century."

Sex: More Than Baby Making

By Nicole Buratti

Physical intimacy strengthens the bond between two people and fosters closeness, love, and affection between couples. It is a major binder that helps couples iron out the differences between them. Physical intimacy builds a stronger connection between two people by mitigating any existing negativity.

Oxytocin, a hormone, and a neurotransmitter, which is released during the intimate moments between the couples, enhances trust and a stronger sense of companionship between couples.

How important is physical intimacy in a relationship, and what does it really mean?

Being physically intimate means more than simply heading to the bedroom with your spouse. Physical intimacy can range from eye-contact, holding hands, cuddling, and of course, sex.

Physical intimacy involves a deep emotional connection that is strengthened when you are in close sensual proximity to your spouse.

Touching, both romantically and otherwise, can help strengthen this bond.

Is physical touch important in a relationship? Yes. What are the benefits of sex? Many.

Having this deep bond can have a positive effect on nearly every other aspect of your relationship.

Infertility is often the first major crisis a couple goes through together. While both partners are impacted, they often deal with the grief of infertility in different ways. Added to the grief is the fact that infertility treatment is expensive and couples often have conflicting relationships to money. All of this drives disconnection. Any disconnection in a relationship will impact its sex life.

Sad but true, it should come as no surprise that couples going through fertility challenges, including treatments such as in-vitro fertilization (IVF), often struggle to keep the intimacy alive. However, never is it more important to have a connection with your partner on both a physical and emotional level. Sex is for pleasure and for reproduction, but attention to pleasure often goes by the wayside for people struggling to conceive.

Often the worst casualty of infertility is the feelings of failure. Sex will often take a turn from hope and connection to a reminder of failure. Once fears of failure or inadequacy enter a relationship, it will drive further disconnection. This will often rupture the secure attachment between partners and the security of the relationship will weaken. Fears of abandonment may even emerge.

The stress of trying to get pregnant can often make sex become more about planning than it is about intimacy. But a lack of sexual activity can lead to emotional instability, relationship problems, and sexual alienation.

A Stanford study documented the extent to which infertility negatively impacts women's sex lives. The study found that forty percent of infertile women suffered from sexual problems that caused them emotional distress compared with the twenty-five percent in the control group of non-infertile women.

While infertility often brings increased depression, anxiety and negative self -esteem, few people talk about how it impacts sexuality. In fact, once infertile, if you want to get pregnant you can't stay in the privacy of your bedroom—reproduction becomes sterile and clinical. What was supposed to be an intimate and private experience between partners now involves doctors, nurses, embryologists and genetic counselors. The intimacy of procreation is now shared with many people at the infertility clinic.

All spontaneity is taken out of sex and couples are often told when they can and cannot have sex. Sex was once a time for a couple to connect and blissfully escape from the troubles around them. It now becomes a painful reminder of the troubles within them.

Women who have a history of sexual abuse or trauma are often re-traumatized by the invasive nature of infertility treatment. They often disconnect from their bodies during procedures and simply "get through" the treatments while holding on to the ultimate hope of conception. Unfortunately, one cannot selectively "shut down." Along with disconnecting from their bodies during infertility treatment, women may shut down the sexual side of themselves.

Even women who do not have a history of sexual trauma may experience trauma from the actual infertility treatments. Your body becomes the focus of scrutiny and many women start to feel shame toward their bodies. They may experience weight gain or side effects that leave them feeling "less sexy." This compounds the feelings of low self-esteem, which will also impact sexuality.

Sex on demand is often stressful for men. It could impact performance. One male client told me, "I never think she wants to have sex with me for me. I think I'm just a sperm machine. Sex has become a means to an end." Approximately a third of infertility is a result of the male factor. While infertility is often a forbidden topic for women, sperm issues are often even more shameful and secretive. When a new dad announces a pregnancy, his male friends will often high-five him and comment, "your boys can swim."

It may seem that since heterosexual couples can only conceive through sex, that it would impact them more than single men and women or same sex partners. However, being able to reproduce is at the core of many people's view of their femininity or masculinity. These feelings of failure and negative views of one's sexual self is pervasive to all who suffer from infertility.

Over the years, I am often asked by clients and even friends, "How to have fun while conceiving." I shared all of the challenges that infertility can bring in the bedroom. But we all want to make fertility fun. They ask, "What are some cool sex positions or creative sexy ideas to make conception exciting?"

Unfortunately, many people lose all sexual identity during infertility. Trying to conceive can often start out fun, however, infertility is simply not fun at all. I realized that as human beings, we are sexual beings and it is imperative that we don't trade our sexuality for our fertility.

How do we get through infertility and find a connection to our sexual selves and our partners while going through infertility?

I have found the following to be helpful:

- Don't wait to address sex until after you have resolved your infertility. People will often tell me that only after they get pregnant and have completed their families, they plan on working on improving their sex lives. This never works. While your sex life may be different during infertility, it does not have to be nonexistent or unsatisfying.

  Consider having sex outside of your "fertile" times to take the pressure off of conception. Avoid only having sex on a schedule. Many couples have told me that once they start infertility treatment, they are relieved to separate sex from conception. Sex can return to being solely for pleasure and connection.

- Familiarize yourself with common challenges that couples face with sex and infertility. Sex is such a private topic so many people don't talk about it. Of course, it is obvious that infertility could impact sex. However, I find that it is helpful to know that you are not alone in this. Also, since infertility treatment impacts such vulnerable parts of ourselves, it is helpful to educate ourselves on what aspects of our lives might be impacted. Joining a support group, online groups, or reading articles can help normalize the impact that infertility has on sex.

- Increase sensuality and spirituality in your relationship. Consider a couple's retreat or spend a weekend at a romantic destination. Take sex off of the table if you are not ready. Cuddle, massage, and hold hands. Remove your fertility books, all injections, medications, thermometers, and notepads, ovulation kits from the bedroom. Take the pressure off of intercourse by expanding your sexual relationship to increased foreplay, erotic touch, role plays (find ways to be sexual with one another without even the possibility of getting pregnant).

- Have an agreement with how much you will share with your friends about your sex life. While it is important to get support, it can be vulnerable and exposing to your spouse if you share details about your sex life without their consent.

- Let go of expectations. There is no right number of times for a couple to have sex. Nor is there one right way. Let go of comparing your sex life to earlier years and open yourselves to sexually connecting in new ways as your relationship evolves.

- Consider seeing a therapist. People may be reluctant to add yet another person into their sex life after doctors, etc., however it is important to address all aspects of infertility. Many people are only willing to treat the medical side of infertility. Therapists that specialize in infertility, sex, and couples therapy could help guide and support you through the isolation and despair that infertility can bring. The couples that seek therapy at the beginning of their infertility treatment fare much better in their relationships compared with the couples who enter therapy after years of grueling infertility with no psychosocial support.

While infertility can be quite traumatic, it can also offer an opportunity for couples. Since infertility is often the first crisis the couple face together, how the couple reaches for one another during this time of crisis can set a tone for the future of the relationship.

While it may be hard to share our deepest and most vulnerable fears of inadequacy and failure, if we can move toward sharing these fears in meaningful ways, it could actually strengthen the couples bond in the long run. Nothing connects a couple more than feeling met and understood during dark times. I find that couples that are willing to share their most vulnerable and scary feelings around infertility are able to secure their emotional bond. When there is a secure bond within the couple, a new and even more connected sexual connection could emerge.

These Are Ten Benefits of Sex In A Relationship.

1) It's an expression of love

One of the biggest reasons why physical intimacy is important in a relationship is because this is one of the foremost ways in which partners express their love for one another. When a relationship lacks sexual chemistry and physical affection, it is more likely to fail.This intimate time you spend together is romantic, thrilling, and releases oxytocin and dopamine. This hormone and neurotransmitter are responsible for feeling closer to your partner, trust, happiness, and even addiction. It's no wonder why physical intimacy is so important in a relationship.

2) Physical intimacy reduces stress

One of the benefits of sex is that it helps minimize psychological stress and anxiety. Being physically intimate in a relationship helps lower blood pressure and reduce stress responses in the brain. And it isn't just sex. Other forms of physical intimacy, such as hugging or hand-holding, can trigger the release of oxytocin.

This hormone will then trigger the brain's reward and pleasure centers, which lowers the feelings of anxiety. One study had participants regularly engaging in intercourse for two weeks to see the effect it would have on stress and anxiety. The results revealed cell growth in the hippocampus, which is the same area of the brain that helps regulate stress.

3) Intimacy with spouse builds trust

Logically, trust is built over time when a couple gets to know one another's true loyalty, patterns, and behavior. But in the heart, or should we say brain, trust is often triggered by the release of oxytocin. Trust is a huge part of relationships.

When two people trust one another, they feel freer to be themselves, aren't suspicious of a third-party entering the relationship, and can be more open, honest, and vulnerable with their spouse. This is one of the benefits of sex too. While having sex or cuddling close on the couch, the brain releases oxytocin, a hormone that makes people more trusting and open to social interactions.

4) Improved intimacy outside the bedroom

The closer you are in the bedroom, the more connected you will feel outside of it. There is a great importance of touch in relationships, and it holds true even for nonsexual intimacy. Being physically intimate with your spouse is one of the biggest ways you, quite literally, connect.

Nonsexual acts of intimacy like holding hands, cuddling, walking arm and arm, and being more physically playful are some loving expressions that come after sex.

Since intimacy raises levels of love-boosting oxytocin and vasopressin, it's no surprise that couples who have sex regularly become more affectionate with one another in other aspects of life.

5) Physical intimacy boosts your immune system

There are benefits of sex, both mentally and physically. Being intimate with your spouse can have a direct effect on your immune system. The immune system receives a boost during sexual arousal and orgasm. When you are regularly sexually active with your partner, you will raise the antibodies in your system that are responsible for fighting against viruses and germs that make you sick.

6) Physical intimacy raises morale

Another importance of the physical relationship is that sex can boost morale.

One study even puts a monetary value on it, suggesting that couples who have sex once a week gain a bigger morale boost than they would if they earned an additional $50,000 a year.

Because physical intimacy in a relationship boosts dopamine, it makes you feel happier. Orgasm aside, one Swedish study suggests that it is the affection that comes before and after sex that offers a boost in morale.

7) It promotes chemistry

Being physically intimate means not only having intercourse with one another but also sharing personal moments of closeness. These can range from a sweet caress, a lingering kiss on the lips, or suggestive proximity. This behavior promotes chemistry and sexual anticipation.

This expectation brings excitement to the relationship and makes couples feel more connected.

8) Health benefits

There are many health benefits that come from being physically intimate with your partner. For example, having sex regularly can lower a man's risk of developing prostate cancer.Being physically intimate without sex also has its benefits. Couples sleep better and feel closer to one another when they cuddle their way to sleep. Oxytocin released by physical touching and sex can also relieve pain and headaches, help you decompress, and reduce many forms of physical illness.

9) Makes you look and feel younger

There may be a correlation between a physically intimate relationship and how young you look. The estrogen and testosterone released during sex may be giving your body a youthful, healthy glow.

Touch is a strong sensation, both physically and emotionally. It brings up feelings of safety, comfort, love, playfulness, titillation, and more. Couples who are physically intimate report a higher rate of relationship satisfaction. When partners engage one another with physical touching, sexual or otherwise, it makes them feel cared about.

Conclusion

How important is physical intimacy in a relationship? Very! Physical intimacy in a relationship means more than being sexually active. It means being emotionally connected. Having a deep connection to your spouse on this level helps build trust, boosts morale, and has many health benefits.

Resources

https://www.fertstert.org/article/S0015-0282(10)00097-X/fulltext
https://www.rtor.org/2019/06/28/mental-health-and-intimacy/
http://journals.sagepub.com/doi/abs/10.1177/1948550615616462
http://journals.sagepub.com/doi/abs/10.1177/0146167216684124

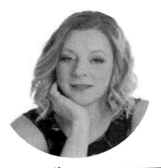

Nicole Buratti
Sex Expert
www.sextalkwithnicole.com

Nicole Buratti is the founder of Sex Talk with Nicole and editor -in - chief of Sex Talk Magazine. She is the author of The GEMMA Method: Sex for the Modern Woman.

Nicole has a passion for celebrating female sexuality and body positivity. She believes that sex is something that should be enjoyed by all women but that it starts with mindset. Great sex has nothing to do with your partner and all to do with you.

Nicole's motto is "Get out (or stay home) and keep it sexy, not for anyone but you."

Nicole is a city girl, born and raised in New York City, who's lived in a bunch of cool places all over the world. Sex,, dating, and relationship advice has always been her jam. She's a girl with a passion and a dream. She's proud to have created her dream.

Nicole has dedicated her life to uplifting women from the outside in by way of the luxury fashion industry and from the inside out when it comes to the holistic model of care. She seriously connects the dots between mind, body, and sexy.

Grit, Grace, Grief, & Joy
By Michelle Byrd

Hey beautiful! Can we just start there? There's nothing more powerful than someone reminding you of how special you are. Going through struggles, especially infertility, can make us forget just how beautiful and amazing we really are.

This project of collaborators came together organically, and I am excited to be a part of it and share my thoughts on infertility. If you're a woman who feels uncertain in your journey and is looking for hope, you're in the right place. If you struggle with "why" this is happening to you, you're in the right place. If you're not sure how your journey will work out, you're in the right place. We are all drawn to this profession for many reasons.

Sometimes, to understand someone's passion for doing what they do, you have to know their "why." I want to start with a small snippet of my complicated journey in hopes that you will better understand who I am, what things I have learned, and to give you something to walk away with when you finish reading this chapter.

I remember lying in bed, with my hand on my belly, feeling the kicks of my miracle twin babies. A boy and a girl, Dion and Layla. IVF success in the first round! And twins! My heart was overwhelmed with joy. All the scary things I had heard about infertility and the IVF process did not apply to me. I did not have to experience some of the nightmare scenarios I had once heard. Everything went so smoothly, and I felt so lucky.

These babies were my dream. I wanted two to three children, but when IVF was recommended, the idea of more than one child was becoming a distant dream. There is no guarantee with IVF. You hope for the best, but it was filled with a lot of unknowns.

I wasn't sure if I would ever be a mother after many months of my husband and I trying on our own. My reality and desperation were that I would be happy with one baby. So, to learn that there were two babies on my first IVF cycle was just a blessing in itself. My family was complete with one pregnancy.

I watched my friends having their children at a younger age and daydreamed about the things I would one day buy for my baby. Let's be real, shopping for babies is so much fun! When I became pregnant, I experienced that shopping for babies was just as joyful as I had always imagined. I ordered two car seats and was always hunting for the perfect nursery items to create the room of my dreams for them – white cribs with everything gender-neutral. I had waited my entire life for this experience and could not have been happier.

It felt that things were finally right in my life after meeting the man of my dreams. I could not wait to share parenthood with him. He was an active duty service member and had many deployments and moves. We were thriving in our careers and were financially stable. The time was right to start our family.

But suddenly, the sound of the nursing station pulled me out of the daydream and reminded me that this time in my life would forever change who I was.

If you remember none of the shenanigans that I write in this chapter, I want you to remember four words. Grit...Grace....Grief.....and Joy. These four things are essential to emotionally navigating your own story.

Grit

What is grit, and what the heck does it have to do with infertility? Grit is passion and perseverance for long-term and meaningful goals. It is the ability to persist in something you feel passionate about and resiliency when you're faced with obstacles (www.newharberinger.com).

Knowing what you want and how badly you want it is the start of knowing just how to use your grit. There will be things that may try to derail your path to building your family, but your grit will keep you on track.

Grit is something that drives you. You may be forced to reflect on your "why" or purpose during your fertility journey, and your grit will be the driving force in what keeps you going. It's the gas in your tank when you're running on empty.

Think about something you really wanted but couldn't have. What was it about your goal that helped you achieve it?

For individuals and couples who want a baby but face infertility, the emotions and stress in the journey have been compared to those experiencing diagnosis and treatment for cancers. Did you hear me? The emotional impact of a life-threatening disease is comparable to the emotional strain of one facing infertility.

Your grit will be your compass when the days are dark. Some may not experience the storm, but wouldn't it be great to always be equipped with what you need IF there is a storm?

Grace

I'm not going to get preachy on you. The grace I reference is the element of movement in beauty or expression.

Isn't that the dream? To move throughout your fertility journey with such beauty and expression? But the reality is, we may move through infertility looking like a broken-down pick-up truck. Stopping and starting, breaking down when things are the worst.

Finding grace during the journey is finding balance in what your journey looks like day-to-day, hour-to-hour, minute-by-minute. You may have had multiple losses or no success in getting pregnant. Balancing all that and gracefully walking through your journey is not something that's done easily.

Being present and focused on your fertility is important. However, not being consumed by it is just as important. You are a person with or without the success of a pregnancy. Your identity of who you are or who you thought you would be will be continually shaped throughout your journey to motherhood. You must have grace, wellness, and balance in your life not to be consumed by the outcome of each phase of your journey.

Grief

First, I want to acknowledge the grief that one may feel just arriving at the doorstep of infertility. There's frustration and sadness with the loss of building a family the way you had always dreamed. Many experience grief initially by unsuccessfully conceiving or when being evaluated and referred for fertility treatment. It's a reality check that your body feels like it's broken.

The strain it puts on relationships is real! You may feel that others just don't get it. Relationships change when you are faced with infertility. Some relationships grow through your experiences, but others may not know just how to support you, including your spouse/partner.

Others mean well but, unintentionally, share comments or advice that is hurtful, which can strain your relationship. This may have you feeling alone.

There's grief when you make major decisions regarding your treatment. Some may not have the financial means to seek IVF, adoption, or surrogacy. Locking away and avoiding these feelings of your grief can be compared to a pressure cooker, which will one day be ready to explode.

Then, there is the loss of the pregnancy that was desperately wanted. That grief is deep and incredibly painful. It should not be compared to the losses of someone who did not experience infertility because they're both great losses.

Your losses and feelings must be validated. You must give space and time for the feelings and the loss that is unique to you and your journey. Many find themselves seeking professional help for their grief, and I couldn't agree more.

Joy

Ahhh...now we've arrived at my favorite...joy. While it may be my favorite, it is the most difficult thing I struggled with during my journey. Through my work in the infertility community, I've learned that many struggle with the same.

I won't sugarcoat it. This is probably the most difficult part of your journey. Joy is what most of my clients need someone to help them with. It's something our brain naturally struggles to comprehend – suffering cannot be parallel to joy.

What do you mean to have joy? I don't have my baby yet!

Having joy does not mean that you have hit the jackpot and have conquered your infertility.

Having joy does not mean that you still do not experience grief.

I don't want you to pretend that you have it all together and that you're not acknowledging and processing the emotions we must all feel in our journey.

Having joy means that you are saving space for hope, while having acceptance for what is, and to live in the moments of joy that come. Some days, you may have to search with a magnifying glass, but the joyful moments are there. I promise.

There's space to be inspired.

Be hopeful.

You are in full control of choosing joy.

I want you to believe in your ability to do anything, even during the hard days.

You will be a whole person in the end, with or without the dream pregnancy you long for.

Being joyful may have you visit the foundation of who you are, your dream, and how you want to experience this dream, even when the road gets bumpy.

Being joyful does not measure your strength or weakness.

We must have time to separate ourselves from the painful path of infertility to prevent us from drowning emotionally. Joy is like your life vest. It's there to always keep you safe from the overwhelming waves that continue to come during your journey. Does that make sense?

Going back to my personal story. You see, when I heard the nursing station sounds while daydreaming with my twins kicking, I was actually lying in a hospital bed at a military hospital waiting for my husband to arrive. My dream had turned into a tragic time in my own journey. Our twin miracle baby boy and girl were going to be born at 18 weeks because my cervix had silently opened prematurely. There were no complications with the babies. They were healthy and thriving.

That night, for the first time in my life, I had given birth to children. My son, Dion, was born first and then Layla, my daughter. They both were alive but died in our arms. We experienced indescribable pain. I still cannot find the words to describe it. We met and said farewell to our beautiful babies in one night.

But I will share one moment that I reflect on from that night. Somehow, through my unimaginable grief, I was able to pause and hold both our kicking babies and say a prayer. I was a mom. That mother instinct kicked in...I wanted to be coherent and have my peace with the way I experienced their passing. I found joy even in that dark moment of losing my babies. That moment changed my grief. I gave my babies to God because it was a part of my values and belief. Having the ability to find that joy gave meaning to their lives.

There were dark days ahead for my husband and I. We got through it with the help and support that was right for us. We sat in the dark some days, but we were never alone. I wish I would have had a fertility coach like myself during my journey. Someone who gets it. A person who would have been there for my husband and I, specifically for the highs and lows when building our family.

If I were anything like Oprah, I would give away babies the way she gave away cars. That show was iconic. Can you imagine...you get a baby... you get a baby...you get a baby!

But the truth is, I can show you how to find joy. No one can promise you that baby. But what I can promise you is the ability to have joy throughout this process if you allow it.

When reflecting on my infertility journey, there are so many moments that could have destroyed me as a person. But they have done the opposite. They have made me a more compassionate, understanding, and loving woman. I found my joy. Baby or not, I was faced with looking myself in the mirror as a complete person. The rainbow baby did come, and I appreciated motherhood differently because I choose to find joy and wholeness for myself during my journey. And you can do the same.

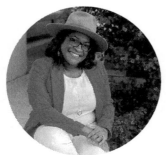

Michelle Byrd

Licensed Clinical Social Worker
www.byrdcounseling.com

I'm Michelle Byrd, a licensed therapist and fertility coach. My mission and passion is to not let others feel broken down from the waves that building a family can bring.

I am a mother, military spouse, and a therapist who has found a way to turn pain into purpose. I love a nice cup of coffee, Netflix, and spending time people in my life.

I have 10+ years of helping people through the things they did not see coming. You know, the life struggles that knock us off our feet and takes our breath away.

The journey into private practice and coaching just felt right to accomplish the goal of being the light of hope for others. Having the right support in place has been instrumental to my own personal growth. I firmly believe that your experience with your journey will be forever changed with the right support.

Turn Every Stone

By Dr. L. April Gago

As REI physicians, our main role is problem-solving. That is what we do.

When it comes to fertility, the first step in problem-solving is identifying the problem, or problems, hindering the desired outcome. This means turning over every stone to ensure the root cause of a problem is uncovered. In the best of times, this presents a rigorous challenge. As with all things, that challenge has been steepened by the conditions of the COVID pandemic. There are more stones than ever to turn.

The Covid pandemic was stressful, and people and entities had to adapt and make changes to the way they do things. My admiration for those who showed agility and creativity under the pressure of Covid soared. The innovative ways people adapted to survive was nothing short of amazing.

In thinking about what makes a strong REI physician, I think it boils down to problem-solving abilities. And the very best have shown the same agility and creativity in our problem-solving abilities as it relates to our work.

I've always felt like REIs are detectives. That it's our job is to listen, look, and find the reasons why conception and live births are not happening for couples and individuals. It's important that we not pull up short. We must turn every stone. Only then do we have the information necessary to devise correct solutions. Only with all answers in hand can we problem-solve to make the changes necessary to achieve conception and live birth.

Some cases are very straightforward and medically solvable. Others are subtle, tricky, and complex. Every case requires the same level of rigor to draw the correct conclusion, and tailor treatment appropriately. Many times there are multiple problems, and sometimes those problems are not easily found. Often the last stones turned reveal the most crucial information.

Talking with people about their lifestyles, including details of their religious, ethical, and personal beliefs can be particularly enlightening. Similarly, probing a patient's sleeping and eating habits, relationship and work struggles, and sexual practices can sometimes reveal issues that weren't previously apparent.

Before this can work, a practitioner must lay a foundation of trust. Only then can the team effort with patients and physicians commence. Certain questions and tests may seem superfluous, and that should be explained, but once trust has been built, patients better accept that it is sometimes multiple small things taken together that unlock the key to fertility. Providing honest and accurate answers to questions and walking through the various tests and evaluations can be crucial to success, and patients who understand the purpose of this process will be more willing to engage.

Once trust has been established, we've been able to address travel, work, and intercourse schedules. We've been able to help craft sleep and exercise schedules for extremely busy professional couples. In this way, we have created opportunities for exercise, meditation, and adequate sleep necessary to foster optimal reproductive health.

Other important components of reproductive health I discuss with patients are diet and supplements. We discuss strategies to improve compliance, time for meal prep, and more. Patients who understand that addressing the seemingly small details that may significantly impact their fertility consistently see better outcomes.

For those who have significant issues with oocyte or sperm quality, uterine factors, or other serious medical issues, it's also crucial to engage in the detailed discussion of options for donor sperm, donor oocytes, donor embryos, gestational carriers, and adoption. Not every patient will initially be receptive to turning these stones, but when placed in the context of the greater goal of achieving the family they so badly desire, they often become more receptive. Removing perceived obstacles and overcoming reluctance to pursue every option for family building is an important step in helping couples move forward with the most appropriate and potentially successful routes for family building.

When treating a couple, it's extremely important to engage both partners. Taking the time to conduct a thorough review of all aspects of fertility for each partner is crucial. Understanding their desires and envisioning a plan for addressing all the potential issues in crafting a design for their family building is my greatest professional pursuit. The greater the complexity, the greater the satisfaction when things go as planned, both for patient and practitioner.

I have families that have worked with my team for months and years to achieve an outcome. With persistence we have been able to succeed in building the family they longed for and feared impossible. This is the most satisfying outcome.

Unfortunately, no practitioner is successful in every case. However, for many patients, persistence and a willingness to pursue many different avenues correlate closely with eventual success. It is these patients who possess the greatest chance of achieving the family they're seeking.

For many patients, the journey is not a direct one. They weather diversions, setbacks, and disappointments along the way. But with persistence, they find the way to the family they're seeking, although the path ends up being different from what they initially envisioned.

Details of what we do can be tedious and burdensome, but when patients understand the process and have the patience to follow the right path, however long or short it may be, they are more likely to be successful. Sometimes more stones are uncovered along the way. We must turn those, too. It's often a stone a bit further down the path that reveals the ultimate solution.

Another important message to patients is to be proactive, but patient. When we recommend diagnostic tests, investigations, procedures, and treatments, it's because we think they will make a difference. Understanding the method to the madness is important. Very often, particularly with patients who have suffered recurrent pregnancy loss (RPL), there is anxiety to conceive again. It's understandable. However, if we haven't figured out the reasons for the miscarriages, pressing ahead too quickly may be counterproductive. Sadly, each miscarriage results not only in additional grief, but also a loss of time while pregnant, as well as having to wait for the passage of tissue, the next normal menses, or even suction D&C procedures. Although these occurrences are safe overall, they can result in potential complications such as uterine scarring if required repeatedly after recurrent losses.

Rather than pushing forward with another conception, it is important to take the time to gather information from the last loss. There are yet more stones that must be turned. Was the embryo chromosomally normal? Is the uterus healthy or are there retained products of conception, uterine scarring, inflammation/endometritis, uterine anomalies, leiomyomas (fibroids), or polyps that could be contributing to the losses? Taking the time to make these determinations before a subsequent conception may prevent unnecessary losses and additional grief and stress.

These tests and procedures can take time, which is frustrating to patients eager for a child, but in the long view, will hopefully lead to information that facilitates the desired outcome of healthy live birth.

I still recommend a series of bloodwork, uterine evaluation, karyotypes for patients considering IVF with genetic testing of embryos, depending on the individual situation. In some cases, certain tests are appropriate for both patients as a couple. Having as much information as possible can be very helpful in moving forward. We simply must take the time to gather it.

Pregnancy success and viability is dependent on a complex series of ongoing events which include good blood flow, proper immune response, a healthy embryo with genetic composition compatible with ongoing development, proper hormonal milieu, including estradiol, progesterone, and healthy thyroxine levels. Adjusting as many of these factors in a favorable direction is the strategy that we utilize to promote ongoing pregnancy and live birth.

In some cases, we note that patients are having pregnancy loss repetitively of chromosomally normal embryos/fetuses, and after elimination of other factors, sometimes a dysfunctional immune response is thought to be the cause.

Before seeing a reproductive endocrinologist/reproductive immunologist I recommend that patients undergo an IVF cycle to create embryos and to ascertain whether the embryos they're using are chromosomally normal, as the woman will be at risk for side effects and complications from the medications utilized during the early pregnancy. If the pregnancy is chromosomally abnormal, the risks to the mother are senseless, as there wouldn't be a live birth with a chromosomally abnormal embryo.

Likewise, testing miscarriage tissue for genetic abnormality whenever possible is also helpful.

Genetic results from previous miscarriages can guide future therapy. I've had numerous young patients with recurrent pregnancy losses that were chromosomally normal (euploid), which gave us the confidence to move forward with other testing and ultimately approach reproductive immunology and immune dysfunction as the etiology for the losses. This assumption can only happen after evaluation for all other potential causes for pregnancy losses have been eliminated. Again, we're turning those stones.

Unfortunately, in reproductive medicine, we struggle to complete large randomized controlled trials, particularly around recurrent pregnancy loss. Due to conditions unique to pregnancy, it's also understandable. It's difficult to design and enroll patients into trials that involve being randomized to either receive or not receive therapy which may be beneficial, or could cause harm, while pregnant. We have some therapies, which while they have not been subjected to objective evaluation in the ideal scientific manner, do seem to provide benefit for some individual patients. As physicians, we must educate patients and help make risks/benefit decisions about which treatments to pursue depending on the circumstances and the overall perceived benefits and risks.

Ultimately, several of these patients have had successful live births with reproductive immunology therapies, but not all. While the successes are encouraging, there is still hope for patients who aren't successful. A gestational carrier or adoption can be ideal solutions to the desire for a family. As stated previously, the greater the willingness of patients to consider all options, the greater the opportunity for eventual success.

Having patients search themselves for the struggles, the things that scare them, and the factors that make them hesitate is helpful. If patients can find a constructive way to share their concerns and reservations, our team can help them find ways to overcome the obstacles they face in pursuing fertility therapies, and ultimately creating the family they long for. Only when you turn every stone do you arrive at the last stone unturned. And it is under that stone that you find a family.

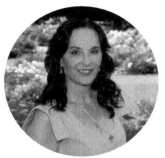

Dr. L. April Gago
Reproductive Endocrinologist
www.gagofertility.com

Laura April Gago MD, is a Reproductive Endocrinology and Infertility Specialist who while on faculty at The University of Michigan, started the donor oocyte program. She then decided that she wanted to provide more personalized, compassionate care. She started Gago Center for Fertility in 2007, and added Gago IVF in 2014, where we provide state of the art fertility care. She is also the founder of Laura's Hope, a nonprofit organization providing financial and grief support for couple who have experienced a loss and are wanting to pursue a rainbow baby.

Infertility and Trauma

By Amy Green

When we are young women, we are storied a narrative of pregnancy and family from our families and society. "First comes love, then comes marriage, then comes the baby in the baby carriage". For 1 in 8 women and their partners, their journey to becoming parents is complicated by infertility. (1) The very fact that we are not able to get pregnant and have a baby with ease can be seen as a reproductive trauma.

Trauma is defined as an event, series of events, or set of circumstances that is experienced as physically and/or emotionally harmful or threatening. This has a lasting impact on the individuals physical, social, emotional, and spiritual wellbeing (2). We see the world differently and experience relationships with people differently after experiencing trauma. It is not uncommon for two people to go through similar life

(1) Cross, C. (2020). Why Can't I Get Pregnant. John Hopkins Medicine. Retrieved from: https://www.hopkinsmedicine.org/health/wellness-and-prevention/why-cant-i-get-pregnant
(2) SAMHSA's Trauma & Justice Strategic Initiative. (2014). SAMHSA's Concept of Trauma and Guidance for a Trauma Informed Approach. HHS Publication No. (SMA) 14-4884. Rockville, MD: Substance Abuse and Mental Health Services Administration.

events and experience it completely differently. For one person, the event could be traumatic, and they could have significant stress responses, and for another they could appear totally unscathed and unaffected. Trauma is truly unique to each person's perception of the event.

With infertility, we can imagine the wide range of events that can be experienced as traumatic. From the medical procedures and hormone shots, to the language that is used to talk about babies. While the goal at the end of the day is to come home with a baby, the means to get to the end oftentimes can be impersonal and traumatic. Another piece to consider is the multiple traumas that can then take place in a person's fertility journey. Here is one woman's narrative to provide an example:

The first time she was pregnant she miscarried at 10 weeks. She was not even scheduled to have an OB appointment until 12 weeks. The second and third pregnancies resulted in early losses as well, with the OB requesting progesterone testing and early ultrasounds to confirm pregnancy with both pregnancies. After the third loss, the client received a bill in the mail from the procedure that was completed at the OB office (DNC) that stated that she had an "elected abortion". She found out that the medical terminology for a DNC is the same as an abortion procedure. This complicated the loss for her significantly, as she felt like her babies were not recognized as babies. She was referred to an infertility clinic where both she and her husband underwent multiple tests to try to figure out why they continued to have first trimester losses. They determined that she would need to go on hormone treatments and do IVF procedures in order to get pregnant and maintain a pregnancy. The clients first round of hormones and egg retrieval failed. None of the eggs had been determined to be viable. The client and her husband did another retrieval, this with a better outcome. The client and husband completed their transfer of the embryo. The first transfer resulted in an ectopic pregnancy where the client had to have one of her fallopian tubes removed. The second resulted in a successful pregnancy and birth.

It is apparent throughout this fertility journey that the client went through multiple traumas, both medical and emotional. Again, this story is starkly different from the narrative that society tells women about their bodies and journey to becoming a parent. This complicates our ability to create meaning, connection, and find support.

Our perception and sensory input can significantly impact whether or not we perceive something as being traumatic. Did we experience something that felt life threatening? Were we scared and confused, with nobody helping to make meaning of the experience for us? Did our bodies feel so out of control that the physical sensations felt scary and overwhelmed our ability to cope? Our interpretation of the world, as well as our understanding of the world, happens through our perception. When we see the people and experiences around us as safe and predictable, our central nervous system is at ease. We feel relaxed, we sleep well, we are able to process information easily, and we can connect.

Infertility can disrupt our ability to feel safe, connected, and can cause havoc on our understanding of our internal sensations. We may not know what is coming next, if the procedure or treatment will work, and much of the situation feels beyond our control. Our internal senses may be significantly impacted by the hormone therapy, procedures, or our emotions. In addition to that, we may find that couples around us do not struggle with becoming pregnant. We may find it difficult to connect with the people closest to us, feeling like we are in different stages and have different stories. We may find ourselves feeling jealous, envious, and sad when we are around friends who maintain these different stories, which complicates our ability to connect further. This can lead us to isolate more so that we do not have to be confronted by the very thing our hearts long for the most: a baby.

Our central nervous system maintains two different responses, parasympathetic and sympathetic. (3) Parasympathetic is oftentimes referred to as the rest, restore, digest response. We are able to sleep well, have our bodies heal well, and have normal rhythms of digestion take place. In this state, we are able to process what we are feeling and make decisions about our responses. So, while we may experience things as stressful, we are able to meet the stress with an appropriate response to help calm our bodies and minds.

With trauma and infertility, we may find ourselves in a sympathetic response. This is oftentimes referred to as the fight, flight, freeze response. We may find ourselves feeling irritable, on edge, and arguing more with those we love. We may notice a significant increase in our anxiety, feel the need to control things around us, or even experience panic attacks. We sometimes even experience disassociation, where we feel detached or checked out of reality. In smaller responses, this can look like spending more time watching Netflix or on social media to check out and detach. In larger responses, this can be truly feeling out of touch and like we are struggling to be present. When we are in a sympathetic state, we also struggle to recall things easily, so we may feel more absentminded or forgetful.

With all of these factors, it is important to find ways to support our bodies and minds with staying regulated. Dan Siegel refers to the ability to stay regulated, the parasympathetic response, as the "window of tolerance". (4) In this space, we are able to respond to stressors without having them overwhelm our ability to cope. Mindfulness is one tool that

(3) Harvard Health Publishing. (2020). Understanding the Stress Response: Chronic activation of this survival mechanism impairs health. Harvard University. Retrieved from: https://www.health.harvard.edu/staying-healthy/understanding-the-stress-response

(4) Siegel, D. (2007). The Mindful Brain: Reflection and Attunement in the Cultivation of Well-Being. W.W. Norton & Company.

we can utilize to support ourselves with having control over how we respond to the situations around us. Mindfulness is the practice of being in the present moment. (5) We can bring present moment awareness to almost anything we do, from mindful eating to mindful walking. This tool helps us to ground in the here and now so we are not worrying over the what if's of the future, or looking backwards at what "should be" and feeling sad or hopeless. There are many benefits to mindfulness, from relieving stress to lowering our heart rate to improving sleep. Mindfulness can significantly improve our reactions to things around us, and when finding ourselves navigating infertility, can allow us to find control over our emotions and reactions, as opposed to feeling out of control. There may be much about the process that is not in our control, but here is where we can find self-agency and be empowered.

There is a paradox at play here. When we have trauma, practices like meditation or some mindful practices can cause us to go to dark places in our minds where we actually exacerbate the anxious thoughts and feelings, instead of supporting them. (6) While we know the long-term benefits of practicing mindfulness and meditation, such as the reduction of stress and anxiety, it is imperative that we bring careful intention and attention to these practices. There are many tools that we can use to ensure that mindfulness is accessible and does not cause re-traumatiziation. Here are a few tips:

- Pick your favorite food to eat and sit down in a place where you feel comfortable and safe. Set a time for two minutes and practice eating mindfully.
- Get in bed with your comfiest pajamas, blankets, and pillows. Notice

(5) Siegel, D. (2010). The Mindful Therapist: A Clinician's Guide to Mindsight and Neural Integration. W. W. Norton & Company.

(6) Treleaven, D. A. (2018). Trauma Sensitive Mindfulness: Practices for Safe and Transformative Healing. W. W. Norton & Company.

the sensations of your pajamas against your skin, feel the different textures of blankets/pillows.

- Sitting on your couch, plant your feet into the floor. Feel into each toe and part of your feet. Take notice of the colors around you. Which colors do you like the most or are the most attracted to? Which colors feel boring or bland to you?

This tool of mindfulness is developed through bringing attention to the present moment over and over again. Are you aware of your body in this moment? Are you aware of your physical self in this moment? Can you feel yourself moving? What feels good in your body at this moment? Where do you notice your breath? Can you bring attention to discomfort in your body without placing judgment on that space? One practice has been written out for you to play with this skill. To truly develop this, you want to do this at least once a day. Start with a minute or two, and over time let it grow into a longer practice.

Remember, there is no right or wrong way to practice this. The key is bringing your attention over and over again back to the present moment. It can be helpful to check in with yourself before and after your practice by asking yourself these three questions:

1) What am I feeling? (name your emotions, happy, sad, scared, anxious, jealous, mad, joyful)
2) How is my breath? (smooth, even, deep, without sound, noisy, rattled, short)
3) How is my body? (relaxed, tense, on edge, tired, exhausted, energized)

Both/And Practice

- Start this practice by finding yourself in a comfortable seated position.

- Begin to bring attention to your breath, slowly being able to notice our inhales and exhales.
- Allow your exhales to deepen and lengthen.
- With each breath, allow yourself to rest in your breath a little bit more.
- Slowly start to bring attention to a place or emotion in your body that feels good, easy, open. See this space and take a deep breath into this place or emotion.
- Notice the sensations that go with this space. Continue to take two more deep breaths in this place or emotion.
- Slowly release and begin to bring your attention now to a place or emotion in your body that feels uncomfortable or even painful. Continue to breathe into this space, as you notice the sensations associated with this space or emotion. Stay connected to this, continuing to take a few more deep breaths into what feels uncomfortable or hard.
- And then slowly start to release this. Bring your attention back now to the place or space that feels good, with ease, and open. Take five deep breaths into this space or emotion. Slowly release from this place or emotion.
- Bring your attention again back to the place or emotion that feels difficult. Continue to breathe deeply into this space, taking five deep breaths.
- One last time bring your attention back to the space or emotion in your body that feels good, easy, or positive.
- Take three deep breaths into this space and feel connected to the sensations of this space. Staying connected to this space of ease, see if you can hold your attention in this space, while bringing a glance over to what feels difficult, painful, or hard.
- Hold about 75% of your attention in the space that feels at ease and good, and 25% of your attention to what feels difficult or hard. Continuing to breathe, notice what it is like to hold space for both, without allowing the difficult or hard to dominate or take over. Take

five deep breaths into this space, continuing to hold space for both.

- When you have finished your final breath, slowly release this practice. Scan your body from the top of the head to the tips of your toes, allowing this practice to settle in your body.

Naming Feelings Practice

It can be incredibly challenging at times to pay attention to the thoughts and feelings we have. Stepping back to observe these thoughts and feelings can prove to be challenging, especially when the feelings are overwhelming and intense. There has been a lot of effective research that Brene Brown (7) & others have promoted around what happens when we name our emotions. To simplify this research, our prefrontal cortex is responsible for decision making, ordering, and what is called "executive function". When we have strong emotions, such as trauma/grief/anger, our prefrontal cortex can become "flooded" or overwhelmed by this emotion, and it checks out. It goes offline. It stops working. The decision-making stops working. So we do not make decisions about how we feel or how we respond to feelings, we just live in the reactions to our feelings. This is where our hippocampus and amygdala come into play. These parts of our brain are more basic in function and they support us in our fight & flight responses. They decide when we are safe (and have emotional and physical responses that follow suit) and communicate to the rest of our body if our heart should race fast, our body tense up, our palms should be sweaty, or if our breath can be deep and with ease.

The concept, "name it to tame it" may sound basic in its function, however, what this has the potential to do internally is quite significant. When we name an emotion or thought, it means that we have to use our prefrontal cortex. Again, when we have strong emotions, this part of our

(7) Brown, B. (2012). Daring greatly: How the courage to be vulnerable transforms the way we live, love, parent, and lead. New York: Gotham Books.

brain is not working to its fullest function. By naming it, we can start to settle our overactive nervous system (amygdala & hippocampus), and re-engage the decision making part of our brain to orient to our emotion so then we can decide how to best respond

For this activity, take out a piece of paper and pen. Set a timer for two minutes. At the top of the paper write down thoughts on one side, and feelings/emotions on the other. Start the timer and begin to write down all of your current thoughts, and then put emotions next to them. See if by naming them you are able to orient to them a bit more, and feel a bit more in control of how you can respond to these emotions.

Closing Thoughts

Mindfulness is an incredible practice and the benefits of this practice can be deeply supportive when navigating infertility. I would be remiss to share with you some gentle reminders for cultivating safety in your mindfulness practice. When we experience big and intense feelings, it can be hard to turn our attention away from them. Mindfulness asks us to tend to the here and now, which can then lead to us feeling triggered, overwhelmed, and re-traumatized when the emotions in the present are distressing due to infertility. Treleaven (8) references many mediation and mindfulness experiences in his book where students and practitioners had the best of intentions going into their practices and were left feeling overwhelmed by their trauma reminders. It is vital to ensure that when our bodies feel overwhelmed and unsafe, we have other places to ground and support us. Some gentle ways to support ourselves in these moments are to have external factors we can attend to. Things such as a palm stone in our hand that we can feel, using tapping or EFT so we can bring sensation to parts of our body, giving ourselves a foot massage, or using

(8) Treleaven, D. A. (2018). Trauma Sensitive Mindfulness: Practices for Safe and Transformative Healing. W. W. Norton & Company.

our sense of smell (such as peppermint or lavender) to support staying present. My hope is that you are able to find spaces of peace in this season.

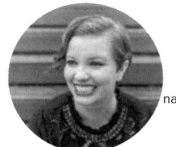

Amy Green, LCSW

Licensed Clinical Social Worker
nashvillecollaborativecounselingcenter.com

Amy Lynn Green, LCSW, ERYT is the Founder and Executive Director of The Rooted Bridge, Owner and Founder of Nashville Collaborative Counseling Center, and it dedicated to increasing access and affordability to mental health support for parents to be and parents across the Southeast region of the United States.

She believes that collaboration in care is a vital aspect to providing support to families. Amy received her MSW from the University at Buffalo with a concentration in trauma informed care and human rights, a certificate from the University of Massachusetts in Integrated Care Management, as well as a certificate in Maternal Mental Health.

Amy works with women and their families, facilitates healing after trauma, supports parents through loss and infertility, and ensures that parents and children have a team collaborating with them in care during pregnancy and into parenthood.

You Are Your Own Medicine

By Lyle Harvey

On this winding journey to your baby, there are many medicines available. Whether you choose IVF, acupuncture, herbal medicine, pharmaceutical fertility medications, functional medicine, meditation, or a combination of many of these, the path that honors your heart and your deep inner knowing is most essential. For it is YOUR unique wisdom and intuition that carry you through the marathon of motherhood.

All of these medicines can have a place in the baby-making journey. Acupuncture and natural herbal medicines are not necessarily the "right" choice in comparison to pharmaceutical medicines. How they are chosen matters. How you interact with your body and emotions concerning these choices changes the overall impact of your fertility journey on your life. Does the journey become a positive "training" experience that increases your confidence in your capacity to mother not only a child with unconditional love and compassion, but also yourself? Or does the journey down the road of fertility treatments leave you feeling like you have lost yourself? Lost your body? Lost your voice and wisdom? Lost your connection to your partner? There is a way to walk through the most invasive parts of IVF and emerge more connected, confident, and alive. There can also be deep healing in turning down the volume of fear and urgent timelines and, instead, tuning into a voice of inner wisdom leading you down a uniquely unconventional, non-medical path. The most fulfilling journeys seem to be those that look a little bit like rocking out alone in your car and dancing to music that no one, except you, can hear.

In my experience of walking alongside many women and couples on this journey, I see the key is becoming your own medicine FIRST. Can you be your own best encourager, compassionate listener, and guide? Think of all the things you long to be in your role as a mother: a comforter, a nurturer, a warm lap, a gentle guide, a giver and receiver of unconditional love, and a cheerleader. Can you give these things to yourself now? You are your own best medicine.

What Is Intuition?

Intuition is called many things: being led by your heart; deep inner knowing; the still, clear voice of your higher self or spirit. Some might associate intuition with not being rational or logical. Intuition bypasses the chatter of the mind, the swirling worries, and endless arguments in your head. Just because this knowledge does not directly reside in the logical mind, which we so value in Western culture, can it still be our truest guide? As children, this inner voice is strong and oftentimes felt on a deep somatic level. Children instinctually know what people in their life feel safe and good. They have no filter and will tell exactly what they feel about everything! Over the years, we learn to be polite, follow the rules, and fit into the crowd. These skills are, of course, important and necessary for us to live peacefully and successfully in community. However, oftentimes these skills take precedence and drown out the inner voice, which always speaks the truth of our wisdom and uniqueness. We've all had the experience of just "knowing" a certain person could be trusted, or one house over another was "The One." However, when it comes to our bodies and proposed medical treatments, many have lost touch with that true voice and knowing. We have been taught to trust the experts. Especially when it comes to the profound longing for a child, most people will do just about anything anyone says to achieve that reality. When women are seeking help from a fertility expert, oftentimes she is already feeling like she and her body have failed to do something that should be "natural." Continuing to trust yourself, your body, and follow your internal guidance system takes great courage. It is vital to preserve this connection to yourself, as this inner knowing is what carries you through all the tough moments of motherhood once that little bundle of joy lands in your arms.

When you are awake with your crying baby at 2 a.m. in a dimly lit room, none of your care providers on your fertility and baby journey are there with you. It's just you and your mama intuition. Your baby is crying. You might be able to easily guess the cause. Maybe teething or reflux? Or it might be completely unknowable with your logical mind. Does this disturbance have a remedy? Need outside help and guidance? Or is this something you cannot completely make better, but your presence and comfort is the right medicine for the moment?

However, when that baby gets into a womb and then gets out of there, the most important thing is whether you emerged from the birthing process of becoming a mother with your sovereignty, your confidence, and trust in your deep knowing intact. All of the other pieces, IVF or natural conception, home birth or hospital, epidural or natural delivery, vaginal birth or cesarean birth, don't govern how you will mother. It's YOU that matters! How are YOU standing in your body? How are YOU feeling in your body? How are YOU speaking to yourself?

Have I seen cases in which a couple has been through multiple grueling, unsuccessful IVF cycles go on to conceive naturally after acupuncture and herbal medicine treatments? Yes. Does this make me the hero of this couple's baby journey? Absolutely not. And if I allow this to be the story, then I am doing these parents-to-be a huge disservice. After being in practice for over 12 years, I have come to see that my greatest gift to anyone who walks through my doors hoping for a baby does not reside in my medical training and licensure. It resides in my ability to guide her back to her own North Star, her inner compass, which is an infallible guide to her baby. This steady voice often resides in the sensations and wisdom of your body, and it will guide you to your next right step. The next step might be deleting social media from your phone, so you no longer torture yourself with the barrage of happy baby pictures. It might be deciding to switch out coffee for a gentler, caffeine-free tea, as you have become aware that the buzz of coffee is leading to poor quality sleep.

Your body will guide and communicate what it needs for your highest good, but are your ears tuned to listen? When your body is allowed to lead, "healthier" lifestyle choices will feel more appealing. These changes will stick much better when they come from a place of inner knowing than when dictated by some expert. This is the process of learning to re-parent ourselves in a gentle, empowered way. Learn to read the signals of your body and heart, and respond to your needs.

I walk a delicate balance in my practice between the roles of healthcare provider and "fertility doula." During the birth process, a doula offers emotional, physical, and informational support so the mother can feel safe and empowered to do the big work of birthing her child. Doula work is often described as "mothering the mother." This mothering energy is not controlling, but creating a safe, nonjudgmental space around the mother in which she is empowered to follow her instincts to birth her child. One of the key takeaways from my DONA birth doula training was not to be the hero and "rescue" a woman from the struggle of her birth experience, but to hold the space for the mother and her partner to emerge from the experience even more bonded to each other and more confident to parent their child. Similarly, when I am supporting women on their fertility journey, I want to make sure that I am getting myself out of the way. It does not serve her and her future role as a mother for me (or any other practitioner) to be the hero, the guru, or the authority. Even if the medicine I am offering is "holistic," if I am offering it in a way that disconnects her from her confidence and wisdom, then it becomes harmful. As a healthcare provider and companion on the baby journey, the greatest gift I can give is to be an encourager of a mother-to-be's intuition and inner-guidance system.

How to Co-Create a Fertility Journey that Honors Your Body and Your Intuition Guide

Choose care providers who will be allies and co-creators on your unique journey. Get clear about what qualities are most important to you. For many women, this list includes things like someone who will listen, takes time to understand your needs, is respectful, knowledgeable, honors informed consent, and has good outcomes. In my experience watching many women go through fertility treatments at different fertility clinics, those who feel seen and heard come out on the other side in a state of greater wellness and balance, physically and emotionally. Even if the process is grueling, consisting of many injections, ultrasounds, and invasive procedures, if a woman can still hear and honor her inner wisdom, she will emerge in a more whole place and ready to mother her child.

Trust the process. Following your intuition does not mean second-guessing and micromanaging all of your care providers' recommendations. It means to choose care providers and helpers from a place of deep knowing, and then relaxing and trusting the process. Sometimes allowing yourself to accept help and care from another can be deeply healing. However, there is a big difference between trusting and checking out. It's important to ask questions. Ask your provider about all of the options, pros and cons, risks, and benefits. This is called informed consent, and you definitely want to find a care provider who makes the time to answer your questions and honors this process. Additionally, it's important to know when something is in your control and when it's not. Once you have chosen your treatment path and provider, the more you can trust the process and embrace the medicine you have chosen, the more your body feels safe and can respond well.

Meditation is not about clearing your thoughts and changing yourself. It is about simply witnessing yourself and what is present for you at this moment. Consciously breathing and witnessing the thoughts passing in mind, like clouds floating across the sky, strengthens one's capacity for being present with what is without judgment. There are countless meditation practices and techniques, including guided meditations that you can download on your phone. To me, the most useful practices are those that strengthen your capacity to have compassion and kindness for your body, emotions, and human experience just as you are. I also love the practice of Tonglen, or Loving Kindness, in which you repeat statements wishing others and yourself well. May you be safe. May you be happy. May you be healthy. May you be free from fear. Sometimes the most seemingly simple practices are the most transformational.

Intuition Strengthening Somatic Practices

Intuition is often most clearly felt on a somatic level. You hear people talk about a "gut feeling" or a "pull on the heartstrings." Our bodies are wise. If you feel pummeled by the tumultuous stormy sea of infertility, it's hard to get your bearings and trust that the ship of your body is indeed equipped with a perfect compass. An exercise I often teach my clients is "Yes and No." Simply place your hands over your heart and begin to breathe. Notice the sensations in your body. Then start repeating the words, "Yes, Yes, Yes." Notice how your body feels. Many people describe "Yes" as feeling expansive, light, or peaceful. Then repeat, "No" at least 10 times. Notice how this feels. People often describe this as feeling more contracted or the sense of a boundary around the body. Yes and No are both necessary. One is good and the other bad. It's important to know what each one feels like in your unique body. This is your inner compass. It is a skill that can be re-learned and strengthened. Try it at first with small decisions, such as what to eat for breakfast or what flavor of tea to drink. Over time, with more practice, you will learn to trust yourself and your intuition more and more.

Nature Connection and Immersion

Sometimes when people ask me what else they need to DO to get pregnant, they want another supplement, herbal formula, or lab test recommendation. Often my number one invitation is to go outside. Find a tree that calls to you. Sit with your spine against its trunk and feel your inhale travel up your spine and exhale travel back down, rooting into the earth. Feel how your breath and body intuitively know how to sync up with the rhythm of this other living creature. Walk outside. Remove your shoes. Let your feet be bare on the earth. Stay until the experience feels complete. This answer can seem infuriatingly simple, but I believe nature is the best teacher for remembering how to be our own medicine. In The Healing Magic of Forest Bathing, Julia Plevin describes forest bathing, which is essentially a practice of mindfulness in nature, as "a process of rewilding, simultaneously the most natural and the hardest thing. It's stomping out all of our learned behaviors so we can reacquaint with our true selves and, with that, the web that comprises every living creature" (pg 2-3).

Every other creature who walks this earth, except humans, gets to enjoy blissful timelessness. They are guided by their instincts to feed

Plevin, Julia. Healing Magic of Forest Bathing: Finding Calm, Creativity, and Connection in the Natural World. Ten Speed Press, 2019.

themselves, procreate, and finding safety and shelter. There is no clock or prescribed schedule. They follow the instincts of their bodies. They read the changing light of the sky, the temperature of the soil, the scent of rain on the horizon. You are made of the same stuff. This rhythm and connection to an abundant ecosystem is your birthright. Allow yourself the gift of timelessness. Charles Eisenstein in his beautiful essay "Initiation to A Living Planet" describes how "a tiny flame of knowledge burns in every person that Earth, water, soil, air, the sun, the clouds, and the wind are alive and aware, feeling us at the same time as we feel them." This exercise is called Earthing or Grounding, which has many scientifically documented benefits, such as direct connection with electrons on the Earth's surface conferring improved sleep, reduced inflammation, a blood-thinning effect, and a shift from sympathetic to parasympathetic tone in the autonomic nervous system (ANS).[1]

However, this medicine is best received not as a prescribed, intellectual exercise, but as an unwinding, a returning, a re-wilding. It is remembering that you are not separate. You are a part of this wild, abundant, fertile ecosystem. An ecosystem that can endure many cases of abuse, toxins, and hurts; yet, if given a moment to rest and breathe, the moss will return. The ferns will bloom again. The earth and all her creatures are designed to regenerate, return to wholeness, and homeostasis. So are you.

Women's Circles

Women's circles can be a powerful way to connect with other women in a non-judgmental environment and reconnect to the beautiful, divine, sovereign woman you are. In the tradition of circles I was taught, we used

Chevalier G, Sinatra ST, Oschman JL, Sokal K, Sokal P. Earthing: health implications of reconnecting the human body to the Earth's surface electrons. J Environ Public Health. 2012;2012:291541. doi: 10.1155/2012/291541. Epub 2012 Jan 12. PMID: 22291721; PMCID: PMC3265077.

a talking piece (as used in many Native American traditions) and only the person holding the piece speaks. There is no crosstalk, no advice giving, no judgment. Each person has time to speak her truth. She comes as she is to the circle and is fully accepted for what she brings in that moment. There is no fixing or rushing in to save someone from their emotions. We listen deeply and stay fully present. We listen without words in our throats. To be witnessed in this way can be profoundly healing and affirming. It breaks patterns of co-dependence of needing others' approval or, in turn, to rush in and try to "fix" someone. The myriad wounds that can be healed and insights that can be discovered through being witnessed and witnessing others in a circle cannot be fully understood until you experience it.

The Path of Co-Creation

In her beautiful book, "The Fertile Female," Julia Indichova describes the fertility journey as "meeting your baby halfway." This concept reminds us that conceiving a child is not just about your body, but also the journey and unique timing of another sovereign soul coming earthside. Depending on your spiritual beliefs, embracing "meeting your baby halfway" can take pressure off of your body and perhaps invite you to dance with the unique soul of your future child until a mutual time and place of earthside meeting is found. Your baby might need to take the "scenic route." Maybe you do too?

The longing for a child is like the rising tide of the ocean. It is irrepressible. That longing is good! Ride that tide of longing to your child. But know that you need not be dragged along the shore, roughed up by the rocks and sand in the process. You can surf that wave with

Indichova, Julia. The Fertile Female: How the Power of Longing for a Child Can Save Your Life and Change the World. New York, NY: Adell Press, 2007.

grace and inner peace. Choose the next right step and then feel your body, feel your breath, feel that surge of longing carrying you forward.

The journey is so much more joyful when you can be your own doula, encourager, and mother. It all begins with being your own medicine.

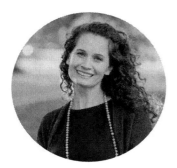

Lyle Harvey

Acupuncturist and
Practitioner of Chinese Medicine
www.nestingplaceacupuncture.com
www.windyacrestn.com

Lyle Harvey, L.Ac, M.S.OM, is a licensed acupuncturist, herbalist and Chinese Medicine practitioner. She holds a B.A. from Wellesley College and a Master's of Science degree in Chinese Medicine from the Seattle Institute of East Asian Medicine. She is a DONA trained birth doula and also has completed advanced training in using acupuncture in labor and delivery. In her private practice in Nashville, she specializes in women's health, fertility, prenatal and postpartum care. She also offers virtual fertility consults, coaching and intuitive healing sessions. One of her passions is teaching meditation and nature-connection practices to individuals and groups. She leads in-person and virtual meditation courses and women's circles.

She lives on Windy Acres Farm, an organic farm near Nashville, TN, with her husband and two children (ages 6 and 3), who were born after a long and winding fertility journey. She personally knows the pain, struggles and unexpected gifts of babies who "take the scenic route" in coming earthside.

Visit www.nestingplaceacupuncture.com to connect with her.

Brain Health

Dr. Kristin Lasseter

Our brain is a very complex organ. It is so complex, we often forget it is even an organ in our body similar to the heart, the pancreas, or the liver. Our brain's function is so important though. Not only does it serve as the conductor of our entire body, but it gives us our thoughts, feelings, memories, and desires. It's the most precious organ we have.

Just like the rest of the organs in our body, our brain can get sick too. Neurons, the cells that make up our brain, malfunction when they get ill. They can stop working the way they normally do. When cells become dysfunctional in the heart, blood is not pumped through the body as efficiently, and certain symptoms arise. When cells become dysfunctional in the brain, they impact thoughts and emotions, as well as how other organs function.

When the brain becomes ill, sometimes we can work hard to change our lifestyle and get our brain healthy again. Sometimes, just changing our lifestyle isn't enough though, and we need medication to help it get back to being healthy. The same with our cardiovascular system - sometimes we can lower blood pressure with diet and exercise alone, and sometimes we need blood pressure medication to help us out no matter how perfect we behave. And there's nothing wrong with that. It's something we cannot fully control - just like most things in life.

When someone suffers from mental illness, their brain is prone to malfunction, whether that's through genetics, development, injury, inflammation, or chronic stress. After a brain has suffered through mental illness, it is then at risk for going back to malfunctioning again in the future. The more times it gets sick, the higher the risk is for future mental illness relapses.

Even when medication is used to help a brain get back to being healthy, medication by itself is usually not enough. Similar to the cardiovascular system, medication can dramatically improve symptoms, but if lifestyle habits are not also improved, the improvement from medication will not be as durable and will not be as effective.

Remember, our brain is complex. We cannot get away with just treating it with medication for very long. Similarly, just doing lifestyle improvements is usually not durable enough to keep a brain from getting ill during increased times of stress. Keeping this organ healthy, just like others, involves using multiple modalities.

So, besides medication, what are the other ways to give a brain the best chance at staying healthy? Similarly, when going through the chronic stress of infertility at a vulnerable age when a brain is most likely to get a mental illness, what can be done to help prevent neurons from dysfunction.

Not surprisingly, the same lifestyle habits that help other organs function well, are the same lifestyle habits that keep a brain functioning well.

Sleep

Sleep is so important. While science has not yet found all of the ways that sleep helps the human body, it has discovered enough to tell us sleep is vital. In fact, without sleep, brains malfunction within days. Without sleep for weeks, a brain can get so ill, that it can cause permanent damage to neurons.

Sleep impacts many areas of the brain that then direct other organs and functions of the body, such as fat composition, stress levels, inflammation, energy, immunity, and metabolism. Those who have chronically disrupted sleep - either from inadequate amounts or poor quality - are at higher risk for heart disease, high blood pressure, obesity, diabetes, dementia, and mental illness. Unsurprisingly, sleep is also correlated with life expectancy.

Sleep is a tricky thing though. It's another one of those issues that we cannot completely control. There is such a thing as worrying so much about sleep, that it causes insomnia. While we cannot have complete control over sleep, we can set ourselves up for getting optimal sleep. Sleep is not the same for everyone, and that's okay too. The most important thing is to practice good sleep hygiene. And, yes, that's a thing.

Exercise

We are all taught from a young age how important exercise is for our body, especially for our heart. However, people are not taught how important exercise is for our brain's function. There are several ways that exercise improves our neuronal function, and so, doing a variety of exercises is likely more beneficial than just sticking to one.

We are all taught from a young age how important exercise is for our body, especially for our heart. However, people are not taught how important exercise is for our brain's function. There are several ways that exercise improves our neuronal function, and so, doing a variety of exercises is likely more beneficial than just sticking to one.

Food

What we eat also impacts the ability of brain cells to function well. Food is a long-standing debated topic in medicine though. There are mixed messages and research out there about what is good for us and what is not. For example, some health experts say we should snack throughout the day, whereas others say snacking one factor that has led to our obesity epidemic. Even the composition of "healthy" food is debated. Fortunately, with the obesity epidemic, research and science have received significantly more funding to understand food and its impact on the body.

There is even research looking at what types of food impact mental health and the brain's function. Again, it is not all too surprising to see that the types of food that are helpful for the function of other organs are also helpful for the brain.

There is an entire field of psychiatry, called Nutritional Psychiatry, dedicated to using food to treat mental illness. That is not to say medication should not be used as well, but Nutritional Psychiatry heavily incorporates food as a fundamental component to healing the brain in mental illness.

Relationships

As humans, we have evolved to be very social creatures. We depend on social and emotional connections with each other to thrive. It could even be argued that we need relationships with others to survive.

There is evidence of the necessity of personal interactions in early infant mental health. Infants who grow up with two mentally healthy parents have higher intelligence scores, better language development, and improved executive functioning than infants who are raised by parents with mental illness. Babies who are neglected or not given adequate attention and affection, are at higher risk for a disorder called failure to thrive. Children who are not socialized with other children through their development have greater difficulty functioning normally as adults in multiple areas. Adults who lack social interaction are at increased risk for severe mental illness.

Essentially, to be healthy at every point in our life, we need social support from other people. The development of the brain is so dependent on those early interactions and relationships, that without them, children are at a higher risk for mental illness, behavioral disorders, and long-term health conditions.

Multiple studies have shown the importance of a woman's support network during the postpartum period, and this makes sense logistically. If a woman has help with cooking, cleaning, working, and taking care of her other children, she is bound to have less stress, and, therefore, is less at risk for postpartum mental illness. Similarly, if she has someone to confide in about her struggles or fears, or someone to give her some time away from her newborn to rest, she is also going to fare better mentally and physically than a woman who does not have those opportunities.

Mindfulness

I will never forget my first patient who struggled with infertility. She was in her second trimester of a very wanted pregnancy, and she was depressed and grieving. This woman had been through so much to be pregnant. She was pregnant just a year prior but had lost her pregnancy in the second trimester. Before that, she had experienced multiple miscarriages and been through a few rounds of IVF.

As she sat on my couch grieving for the baby she had lost a year before, my heart broke for her. How could someone endure so much? How could they find the strength to try again? More importantly, how can they heal from all of the trauma to be there for their growing baby? Over the years, I have realized such determination to have a child was not unique to this woman. It seems more common than ever to see couples going through infertility and hoping to have a child of their own. They fight through obstacles and demons to make their dream come true. It's love and determination unlike anything else in this world.

The expectation for the journey of trying to have a child can be a double-edged sword. On one side, it provides hope and hope is a powerful thing. On the other side, it has an element of trying to control the situation. Fertility is not in our control though, and the more one tries to control it, the more frustrated one becomes. Expectation is best held loosely. Life never goes according to our plan. Life is only made up of moments. Moments we often have no control over. If we don't try to revel in the present moment, then it gets harder to appreciate life the longer it goes on. Even when our dream finally does come true.

It is important to live in the moment. But, how do we live in the moment when we spend our lives working hard toward a goal? We end up spending every moment with our thoughts in the future planning how to accomplish our dream, or with our thoughts in the past figuring out what we did wrong and how to learn from it. While this is a great way to accomplish goals, it doesn't leave us with much value in the present moment we're living. Once we make it to that goal or our dream finally comes true, we have forgotten how to stop and enjoy life. Instead, our thoughts are somewhere else. Thinking about another dream, reminiscing, or worrying about losing what we have.

Life is only made of moments, and the only moment we can experience life in is the present one. If we're rushing through those moments, we're not living life. Being present in the here and now has been shown to be so beneficial to the health of our body. Research has shown the structure of our brain actually changes with regular mindfulness practice, and perhaps these changes are what cascade through the body to improve aspects of physical health as well. After all, mental health is one of the most important factors in maintaining physical health.

Mental health is also one of the key factors in raising happy, healthy children, but taking care of our mental health can feel selfish. Somehow our culture has put mental health near the bottom of the totem pole of priorities. Our mental wellbeing does not just affect ourselves though, it affects those we closely interact with too.

Staying in the moment - healthier mental wellness - better parent - more thriving child.

So for you, for your loved ones, for your future loved ones, stop. Stop waiting for what's to come. Stop dwelling on what's been lost. Stop trying to be better, and - Just. Be. Here. Now.

The research content from this chapter can be found in the following sources:

1) Cappuccio FP, D'Elia L, Strazzullo P, Miller MA. Sleep duration and all-cause mortality: a systematic review and meta-analysis of prospective studies. Sleep. 2010;33(5):585-592. doi:10.1093/sleep/33.5.585
2) Fung, Jason. The Obesity Code: Unlocking the Secrets of Weight Loss. Vancouver: Greystone Books, 2016. Print.
3) Goel N, Rao H, Durmer JS, Dinges DF. Neurocognitive consequences of sleep deprivation. Semin Neurol. 2009;29(4):320-339. doi:10.1055/s-0029-1237117

4) Jenkins DJ, Wolever TM, Vuksan V, Brighenti F, Cunnane SC, Rao AV, Jenkins AL, Buckley G, Patten R, Singer W, et al. Nibbling versus gorging: metabolic advantages of increased meal frequency. N Engl J Med. 1989 Oct 5;321(14):929-34. doi: 10.1056/NEJM198910053211403. PMID: 2674713.

5) Patel A, Sharma PSVN, Kumar P. Application of Mindfulness-Based Psychological Interventions in Infertility. J Hum Reprod Sci. 2020;13(1):3-21. doi:10.4103/jhrs.JHRS_51_19

6) Kumagai, N., Tajika, A., Hasegawa, A. et al. Predicting recurrence of depression using lifelog data: an explanatory feasibility study with a panel VAR approach. BMC Psychiatry 19, 391 (2019). https://doi.org/10.1186/s12888-019-2382-2

7) Li J, Long L, Liu Y, He W, Li M. Effects of a mindfulness-based intervention on fertility quality of life and pregnancy rates among women subjected to first in vitro fertilization treatment. Behav Res Ther. 2016 Feb;77:96-104. doi: 10.1016/j.brat.2015.12.010. Epub 2015 Dec 19. PMID: 26742022.

8) Novotney, A. (2020, March). The risks of social isolation. Monitor on Psychology, 50(5). http://www.apa.org/monitor/2019/05/ce-corner-isolation

9) Ramchandani P, Stein A. The impact of parental psychiatric disorder on children. BMJ. 2003;327(7409):242-243. doi:10.1136/bmj.327.7409.242

10) Ramsey, Drew. Eat Complete: The 21 Nutrients That Fuel Brainpower, Boost Weight Loss, and Transform Your Health. , 2016. Print.

11) Rowland TA, Marwaha S. Epidemiology and risk factors for bipolar disorder. Ther Adv Psychopharmacol. 2018;8(9):251-269. Published 2018 Apr 26. doi:10.1177/2045125318769235

12) Schuch FB, Vancampfort D, Richards J, Rosenbaum S, Ward PB, Stubbs B. Exercise as a treatment for depression: A meta-analysis adjusting for publication bias. J Psychiatr Res. 2016 Jun;77:42-51. doi: 10.1016/j.jpsychires.2016.02.023. Epub 2016 Mar 4. PMID: 26978184.

13) Sim K, Lau WK, Sim J, Sum MY, Baldessarini RJ. Prevention of Relapse and Recurrence in Adults with Major Depressive Disorder: Systematic Review and Meta-Analyses of Controlled Trials [published correction appears in Int J Neuropsychopharmacol. 2016 Apr 27;:]. Int J Neuropsychopharmacol. 2015;19(2):pyv076. Published 2015 Jul 7. doi:10.1093/ijnp/pyv076

14) Vaezi A, Soojoodi F, Banihashemi AT, Nojomi M. The association between social support and postpartum depression in women: A cross sectional study. Women Birth. 2019 Apr;32(2):e238-e242. doi: 10.1016/j.wombi.2018.07.014. Epub 2018 Sep 28. PMID: 30274879.

15) Zhao Z, Zhao X, Veasey SC. Neural Consequences of Chronic Short Sleep: Reversible or Lasting?. Front Neurol. 2017;8:235. Published 2017 May 31. doi:10.3389/fneur.2017.00235

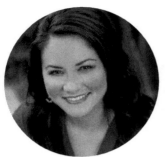

Dr. Kristin Lasseter
Reproductive Psychiatrist
www.rpcaustin.com

Kristin Yeung Lasseter, MD is a Board Certified Psychiatrist in Austin, Texas, who specializes in Reproductive Psychiatry and Women's Mental Health. She attended medical school at the Long School of Medicine where she was awarded membership into the prestigious Alpha Omega Alpha Medical Honor Society, and completed Psychiatry residency at Dell Medical School at The University of Texas where she served as Chief Resident.

Dr. Lasseter received additional training in Reproductive Psychiatry at Baylor College of Medicine prior to starting Austin's first Women's Psychiatry clinic in her fourth year of residency, and was awarded the Association of Women Psychiatrists Symonds Fellowship for her efforts and dedication to advancing Women's Mental Health in Central Texas.

Dr. Lasseter started Reproductive Psychiatry Clinic of Austin in 2018, which hosts multiple psychiatrists and psychotherapists specializing in mental health encompassing the reproductive life span. Additionally, she provides perinatal consultation to one of Texas's busiest women's hospitals, is the Medical Director of the Pregnancy and Postpartum Health Alliance of Texas, and serves on the committee for the Texas Perinatal Mental Health and Wellness Conference.

Dr. Lasseter volunteers much of her time to raising awareness about reproductive mental health to the public and to other medical providers through speaking engagements and social media.

The Fertility Journey

By Michelle Oravitz

After working with many couples who struggled to start a family, I have learned that the fertility journey is anything but linear. Couples endure months or even years of testing in hopes to uncover the obstacles that have prevented them from actualizing their dream of becoming parents. They experience conflicting emotions as they witness their friends and family effortlessly start families, not knowing how to be happy for those who they love while feeling defeated at the same time. To make matters worse, after what seems like endless tests, many couples are told that there is no medical explanation for why they can't get pregnant!

As a practitioner of Oriental medicine, my first goal in helping my patients is to bring harmony in every aspect of their lives. When I first sit down with my patients, I explain to them that reproductive health will always reflect overall health. Approaching the body to simply get pregnant will not produce the desired outcome unless it is understood that the main objective needs to start with the foundation – which is overall health and vitality. We hear about "balance" often, but what does it even mean? I will go over exactly what it means and why it is often used in TCM or Traditional Chinese Medicine.

Chinese medicine is an ancient form of natural medicine that has been practiced for at least 3,000 years. The actual dates are unknown because many books and materials have been lost from events such as book burning by certain governing bodies throughout history in China. TCM has its roots in Taoism. The main idea behind Taoism is that if we live by the way of the "Tao", which translates as "the way" or way of nature, we will be free of suffering, disease, and disharmony. "The way" reflects the natural balance of harmony that is observed in nature. Nature is designed to self-harmonize and works effortlessly to create this balance. The sun provides heat but is balanced and kept in check as night arises and cools down the earth and plants. All "parts" in nature are used as a perfect puzzle to work together as a "whole". Even manure has the purpose of fertilizing the soil to help grow new life. Nature is designed like an eloquent symphony harmonizing itself at all times. We as humans are part of this amazing nature and are also designed to self-heal and harmonize.

The Balance of the Yin and Yang

A symbol that visually describes the harmonious balance that Traditional Chinese Medicine refers to is the yin and yang. The yin and yang is a symbol of a pair of opposites working together to keep each other in check. Just as night transforms into day, Yin transforms into yang and just as day transforms into night, yang transforms into the yin. Yin has qualities that can be described as moist, cool, dark, feminine, passive, slow, and inert. Yang has qualities that can be described as dry, hot, bright, masculine, active, fast-moving, and dynamic.

Everything on earth has elements of yin and yang. If you look at the yin and yang symbol, you'll also notice that it has a small circle of the other on each side. They not only transform into one another, but they embody a hint of one another as well. All living things have opposite forces within them. The two opposites working together support life.

94

Women and men are a perfect example. The two opposite sexes coming together support a new life. The sperm is very yang and active, yet it is surrounded by moist semen which is very yin to protect and help it travel. The egg is very yin as it travels slowly and is stable, but it also has a ton of mitochondria which are yang energy powerhouses ready to get going when it fertilizes with the sperm! This is the beautiful harmonious design of nature – and it is designed with balance in mind.

Homeostasis is the term used in science that pretty much sums up the yin and yang! Homeostasis is what causes FSH to rise if the ovaries don't respond as fast. We have our internal thermostat and detection in our bodies to let the body have extra or less of something to create homeostasis. What's amazing is that the body is speaking to us all the time! It tells us when we're hot, cold, hungry, tired – all to signal us to change our behavior so that we can quickly correct whatever imbalance the body is detecting. If we are so perfectly designed, why then, are we experiencing imbalance?

Living in Disharmony

We are living at a time where we get rewarded for ignoring our needs. To get that promotion, get the best grades, or look our best (to name a few), we need to stay up when we're tired, sit for prolonged periods, skip meals when we are hungry, over-exercise, and the list goes on. We have been conditioned to believe that ignoring our body's cues is not only perfectly fine, but it will also get us what we want. We deprive ourselves so much of proper nourishment and then swing to the opposite extreme of over-eating. We deprive ourselves of sleep and find ourselves never finding a moment when we feel energized. Even imbalance has a yin and a yang aspect! We flip from one extreme to the other because our bodies are screaming for balance.

Not only is this a behavioral issue, but we are also bombarded with outside toxins that influence our delicate hormonal and health balance. Our food, cosmetics, pesticides, cleaning products, containers, may have ingredients that disrupt our hormones and reproductive health. These add to some of the factors that contribute to our overall disharmony. Although we can't altogether avoid many of these, we can educate ourselves and choose products that are safer for our overall health.

Another contributor to living out of balance is how we think, feel, and act. Our mindset can have a very powerful impact on our health. When watching television, we enter a state of trance similar to that of hypnosis. Watching disturbing events on the news adds to our feeling of anxiety and puts us in a state of fight or flight. Anxiety and stress do not help the reproductive system. Our bodies respond to a feeling of fear by shutting down functions that aren't essential for survival.

Living in disharmony is living out of alignment with what is in our well-being's best interest. When we are aligned, life feels effortless. Alignment means learning to listen to your body and intuition and be guided to eating the right foods, living a life that feeds your soul, mind, and body, thinking empowering thoughts, and spending time with people who uplift your spirit. These are things that make us feel good and they do so for a reason. Our feelings and sensations are a barometer of how aligned we are in our lives. Again, the nature that designed us is so intelligent. Luckily, it is also very simple.

A Return to Harmony

Returning to harmony has to start with one step – awareness. Awareness is the first step to uncovering where we are experiencing disharmony. It is important to point out that there is a distinct difference between something common and something normal. An example of this is something that I used to believe before studying Chinese medicine, and this was that PMS was normal. After studying Chinese medicine, learning the patterns that contribute to PMS, and seeing myself and my patients have monthly cycles with no PMS symptoms, I was awakened to this amazing realization. As a collective, we experience many common symptoms and ailments due to shared contributing factors such as environments, habits, toxins, and cultural behaviors. When we have these shared imbalances, they start to appear as normal and we accept them as simply part of life.

When we begin to practice awareness and become mindful of our well-being, we can address any changes that need to take place that will restore us to balance. The beautiful thing about restoring balance is that it can be addressed in many different ways. If you learn to master just your mind, you can evoke miraculous healing for not only your body but your entire life. This includes relationships, mental well-being, health, and alignment with your life purpose. I believe that if we ignore something such as the work you do daily, you may be ignoring a major contributing factor to your imbalance or symptoms. Our emotional harmony directly affects our physical health, and it is important to finally look at our health as an all-inclusive aspect of our lives.

Awareness can be practiced by taking a few minutes a day to get quiet. Doing so may seem like nothing is happening, but the opposite is true. When we take time to get still in a consistent practice of meditation, we are allowing ourselves to tune into a state of receptivity. This is a state of listening that re-trains our minds to connect to the subtle sensations of our bodies. As mentioned earlier, our body signals us to know what it needs to maintain homeostasis or balance. The more we allow ourselves the opportunity to listen, as in the state of meditation, the more unmistakable our body's cues will become. Taking the time daily to sit in stillness will not only allow us to connect with our ability to discern our body's language, but it will also create a state of relaxation that encourages mental and physical restoration.

This state of relaxation is another very important step to harmonizing the body. One of the ways that acupuncture helps the body's ability to heal, is by creating a state of deep relaxation. When we are in this state of relaxation, our body's ability to restore itself becomes more effortless. A term used to describe this state is "Wu Wei". Wu Wei is a Taoist term that refers to the effortless effort we see often in nature. As Lao Tsu beautifully said, "Nature does not hurry, yet everything is accomplished". A bird feels the urge to fly so she flaps her wings, when she reaches the right height and feels the wind, she surrenders and allows herself to be flown by the wind. It's this knowledge of when to exert and when to let go that is reflected in Wu Wei. By letting go and allowing the body to surrender, tremendous effort can take place among the cells and bodily systems to heal and restore the body. This is a beautiful example of yin and yang embodied.

Getting into a state of both awareness and surrender allows us to be guided towards our path to well-being. I have met many women through my podcast who have set on a detective quest to figure out why they weren't able to get pregnant. They investigated through many different means such as charting their cycles and daily basal temperatures, observing their cervical mucus, starting an elimination diet, and speaking to many different professionals to get to the bottom of why their bodies weren't able to conceive. Many of them (in hindsight) thank the challenges that forced them to listen and learn what their bodies were asking of them.

How you can invite balance into your reproductive health?

Now that you understand the basics of yin and yang and why it is so important for your overall and reproductive health, here are some tips you can do to jump-start your healing process. Before starting any new lifestyle regimen, you must speak to a qualified physician about your current state and investigate to be sure that there aren't any serious underlying conditions that are preventing you from getting pregnant. Feel free to either use all of these tips or just the ones that speak to you. Everyone resonates differently with different methods of healing, so be mindful of what feels aligned for you.

My first suggestion is to begin a daily regimen of charting your cycle and recording your daily temperature with a basal body thermometer. This is a special thermometer that can be purchased online and is not the same as regular thermometers. It is important to be sure to track it every morning before you get out of bed, and ideally after at least three consecutive hours of sleep. It is also best if this is done close to the same time every day, but it's better to have inconsistent hours than to let that goal stop you from doing this altogether. You can print out charts and do this on paper or use apps such as Kindara or Glow. These apps also have questions that you can enter throughout your cycle such as how your feeling, what your bleeding is like during menstruation, and when you notice cervical mucus.

Doing this is one of the steps you can take to increase your awareness. Taking time to notice how you feel and what is happening throughout your cycle is a practice that will get you to pay attention to many subtleties that you may have not noticed in the past. I like to refer to this as engaging in a mindful cycle. I also suggest becoming mindful of your body sensations throughout the day. You can even carry a journal with you throughout the day and jot down how you feel after eating certain foods, spending time with certain people, doing work, exercising, and so on.

My next suggestion is to create a meditation practice. Many people are hesitant or feel that it's too challenging to get a meditation practice going. I have a very simple trick to help. For any habit to start, we need repeated behavior. Many think that they need to start with twenty minutes per day of meditation and that usually doesn't work because it's too tall of an order. I say start with five minutes every day just to start the habit and to convince your mind that this is a new routine that you are adopting. After you get used to the routine you can extend the time. Another thing to keep in mind is that meditation is not the practice of stopping your thoughts – this is a common misconception that can be very discouraging because it's an impossible expectation that even the most seasoned meditators don't do! Common meditations include awareness of the breath or repeating a mantra in one's mind.

The idea of meditation is to be aware of your thoughts with curious observation while favoring awareness of the breath or mantra. Over time, this will retrain your mind to loosen its attachment to the thoughts and instead become more present. The benefits of meditation cannot be underestimated. Creating a practice that induces calm has tremendous benefits not only for our mind and body, but it has also been shown to benefit fertility health. In a study led by Dr. Alice Domar, 54 women who completed a behavioral treatment program based on applying a relaxation response showed that they not only experienced a decrease in depression, anxiety, and fatigue – but 34% of the women in the study also became pregnant within six months of completing the program. https://pubmed.ncbi.nlm.nih.gov/2078200/

Another great way to evoke balance within our body is to connect with nature. TCM views the body as a microcosm of the environment. Nature is beautifully cyclical and can be utilized as a natural entrainer – meaning that by syncing with nature we may be able to also harmonize our internal bodily systems. I often suggest for my patients to take time to ground their bare feet on the earth, only if the weather is warm enough and not during cold weather. Another suggestion I have is to get sunlight in the morning when the sun is safest (unless it is winter and it's safe to get it during the day). Getting sunlight will help synchronize the circadian rhythm and will also help encourage melatonin production, which is an important hormone for sleep and egg quality.

Apart from getting sunlight, I also suggest to get your nightly dose of moonlight! Many women tend to have their cycles entrain with the moon. Most women get their periods during the new moon and ovulate with the full moon, while some are referred to as "blood mooners" and get their periods with the full moon while ovulating with the new moon. Neither one is better, but it is beneficial to allow the eyes to gaze outside at night to synchronize with the natural cycle of the moon. Another very important thing to be mindful of is the amount of artificial light you are exposed to at night. Allow for some time of dim lights for an hour or two before going to sleep, avoiding any screen time.

The key point to remember is that our bodies are designed to "favor" balance. They work to move in the direction of healing at all times. If you want to improve your fertility, the first step is improving the overall health of your body and mind. Although we have been conditioned that we need to work hard to get what we want, it is actually in the state of effortlessness that we are guided to eating the right food, experience more ease, and allow for balance to occur more easily in our health and lives. After years of working with women who have had their hope crushed for many years only to turn their lives around and finally conceive – I have a deep faith in the body's miraculous ability to heal itself.

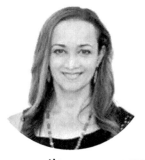

Michelle Oravitz
Acupuncturist
www.michelleoravitz.com
www.thewholesomelotusfertility.com

Michelle Oravitz is an acupuncturist specializing in fertility health, who decided to change her career from architecture to natural medicine in the early 2000s. It was not until her life was transformed by acupuncture, that she was inspired to change her path. Michelle suffered from missed periods from the time she was thirteen. After years of being prescribed birth control pills by Western medicine doctors and then coming off the pill to continued missed periods, she decided to go to an acupuncturist named Dr. Li who immediately regulated her cycle.

It was this transforming event that inspired her to learn Ayurveda and later Traditional Chinese Medicine. She also realized that had it not been for Dr. Li, she would have struggled for many years to get pregnant. This realization, coupled with a natural fascination to learn about fertility drew her to specialize in fertility wellness. She is passionate about empowering women and couples to take ownership of their health and well-being.

Her method of treatment encompasses not only herbs and acupuncture, but also incorporates hypnotherapy, diet, supplements, essential oils, and most importantly, the mind and how it influences conception. Michelle helps women and couples conceive both in person and virtually.

Michelle is the host of 'The Wholesome Fertility Podcast' where she features leading professionals from the fertility world and shares her own fertility wellness tips with her listeners.

Thrive

By Cathie Quillet

"Promise me," he said.

I sat up as the ultrasound tech showed herself out of the room. Broken and in that stale, paper gown, I stood up and fell into his arms. Stabilizing the both of us, his tears spoke of the deepest heartache. He squeezed my cheeks and looked into my soul.

"Promise me," he said. "Promise me this isn't going to change us."

Pregnant, we walked into that room where excitement met pain. Carrying a heartbeat-less baby, we walked out.

Hand-in-hand, into the most devastating of situations, we walked past the hopeful parents, the unassuming every-dayers, and those who hadn't just experienced their world falling off of its axis.

It was just us now.

Infertility and pregnancy loss are situations that put you at the crossroads of your relationship. Do you merge together or do you start walking independently? Do you lean into each other or into support systems external to your relationship? Do you become more one or does the oneness of your relationship start to become two again?

My depths of despair looked like endometriosis, PCOS, adenomyosis, recurrent pregnancy loss, permanent barrenness, and a hysterectomy at thirty-two.

I wonder what tragedy, or what we now call a reproductive trauma, brought you to your knees. I wonder what bookmark moment intersected with your mundane and taught you grief. As that moment comes to recall for you, here is my question to you:

What Did You Auger In To?

I am a reminiscer by nature. My favorite story growing up was my mom's birth story with me. Every time that we were alone, I would ask her to tell me the story of when I was born.

Holidays, New Years', anniversaries, and most days in between cause me to reflect. What was the story? What was the lesson? How did I grow? Who did we become out of it?

I remember driving the long and congested streets of Toledo, Ohio when my husband and I were going on a date to celebrate our anniversary. As I reflected on our years together, I asked him, "What are the highlights for you?" Of course, the moments and memories that filled our scrapbooks were recalled; but there were two answers that completely shocked us.

My answer: Infertility.

His answer: Our miscarriages.

Our why's were the same. Without those hellish experiences, we would not be the couple or the individuals we had become as a result.

We grew and had the emotional stretch marks to show it. We fought for unity and continued to show up for each other and for our relationship. In the midst of the struggle, when the waves crashed around and our boat threatened to capsize, our foundation felt murky.

But then came the rising. The growth. The togetherness.

Infertility

For the seven-in-eight of the population, saying the word infertility means not having a baby. It means more opportunities to have sex and the postponement of sleep-deprived nights and poopy diapers.

For the one-in-eight of us, we know that infertility means a lot more.

It means standing on the outside of social circles contemplating our current identity in them, wondering when we became less of a woman than those still inside the circle.

It means still being in or close to the honeymoon phase of your relationship, dreading the connective act of sex because it probably is just going to yield another negative pregnancy test, and wondering if you can handle it.

It means not knowing what the date is but knowing what cycle day it is and what medicinal intervention is coming next.

It means wondering if your partner would be better off with someone with a functional uterus, better sperm quality, or healthy eggs.

It means heartbreak, depression, apathy, anxiety, and crying in public, in private, and without even being aware tears are streaming down your face.

Let's talk about some prescriptions that can help you thrive in the midst of this heartache.

Team Marriage

I always tell my clients that I think there are three people in a relationship.

You, your partner, and your relationship.

Here is an example of what I mean: If you and your partner are fighting about something and you going into it feeling like you need to "win," then your partner and your relationship lose. If those two lose, sorry to say, but you do as well.

If you and your partner are fighting and you are on the side of team marriage, meaning that you're not out to prove your point, belittle, or shame, then your partner, your relationship and you win.

Here's how this works during infertility:

Partner 1: "Honey, I am really sad about everything. This is all too much. I feel like I'm going to break."

Partner 2: "I know, you have said that before. I can't talk about this anymore. It's all we ever talk about."

That is NOT team marriage.

Let's try again.

Partner 1: "Honey, I am really sad about everything. This is all too much. I feel like I'm going to break."

Partner 2: "I know this is so hard, babe. I hate it too. I know how much you hate sitting in these difficult emotions. What can we do together to bring you out of this?"

Do you see the difference there? Example one is me-centered. Example two is us-centered. It's solution and relationship focused.

In the midst of grief, pain, and situations that feel too difficult to overcome, think: "Am I on the side of team marriage, or am I out for myself?"

In other words: "Can we grow positively out of this or am I doing damage to the relationship?"

At the end of every disagreement, fight, or impossibility, it is my firm belief that we ought to be better on the tail end. That is team marriage.

Friendship

When we're new in a relationship, our focus is romance, deepening our emotional intimacy and flirtation.

When my husband and I were dating, we spent hours talking on the phone playing the let's-get-to-know-you game. We were intentional on our dates, maximizing our minutes together, and longing for each other while we were apart.

When was the last time that you and your partner did anything that looked like flirting or romance?

Without the trauma of infertility, as the years count on, friendship takes the back seat to "did you do the dishes?" And flirting? That takes the back seat to chores, work, and the business of doing your life together.

I recall a meeting with a client who I'll call Roxanne. She sat across from me, lamenting about the emotional distance between her and her husband. She spoke adoringly about their early years of marriage, juxtaposing them against her current feelings towards their relationship. "I feel like I don't even know him anymore."

They were in the midst of grief together but were processing it so very differently. He plugged in, to video games, gambling apps, and the mundane scrolling of social media. In response to his avoidance, she found her refuge in her support groups and anyone that seemed to express concern about their story.

As the negative pregnancy tests collected in the wastebasket, so did their relationship. They initially went to doctor's appointments together and then they didn't. They spilled tears together and then they stopped all communication about infertility, emotions, and anything more than who paid the bills and when upcoming appointments were. They were emotional strangers.

"What if you went on a date?" I asked.

"What would we even do?"

"What did you do when you were dating?"

"We loved kayaking," she said.

Start there. Not in conversations or repair.

Start in recalling the friendship that brought him to one knee and you to the white dress. Find the muscle memory of the friendship.

I remember one August afternoon, my husband and I were driving back to Ohio from a Detroit Tigers baseball game. We had spent all day in Detroit, eating, taking in batting practice, and watching his favorite team.

On the way home, I said, "I missed you today. When we get home can we spend some time together?"

Baffled, he said, "We were together all day."

He was right but we were shoulder-to-shoulder. We didn't talk about how anything felt, what we enjoyed, or anything below the surface.

While I loved our shoulder-to-shoulder time, I craved some face-to-face time. I wanted to talk about something other than baseball, BBQ, or batting averages.

When I suggest that you explore your friendship and jump in your proverbial kayak, I am suggesting some shoulder-to-shoulder time. Start there. Find what you used to enjoy and then work back into the emotional intimacy, just like you did at the beginning of your relationship.

Deepen Emotional Intimacy

Picture an iceberg with me. We can all thank the movie "Titanic" for educating us about icebergs, can't we.

Emotional intimacy deepens as we dare to go below the surface.

We can have shallow conversations with those in the grocery store, lunchroom, or church lobby. "Hi, how are you?" "Good, how are you?" Walk away. It's over.

Just below the surface of our emotional iceberg, you may have depending conversations with cubicle mates, your in-laws, or some friends. "Hi, how are you?" "Boy, am I tired. It was a long weekend. How are you?" It feels surface but looks a little bit deeper than our first example.

At the depths of our emotional iceberg lives only what you want to admit to yourself. Vulnerability lives here. Sacred memories, experiences, and emotions live here. Share it with someone if you dare. That is intimacy.

I remember our third miscarriage, standing in the checkout line of our local grocer. "How are you today," the politely unassuming woman asked.

"How am I doing? I have a dead baby in me and it isn't the first. I can't carry a baby to term like everyone else in this baby-breading land seems to be able to. I'm broken, depressed, and alone. How do you think I am?"

Of course, I didn't say any of it.

"I'm good," I said as I paid for the supplies I thought I would need to carry out the miscarriage at home. "How are you?"

While I wouldn't dare share what was really going on in my heart, someone with whom I had a deeper emotional intimacy could have shouldered the ache of my heart.

While you and your partner may be experiencing different emotions at different times, connection here is key.

Days before my twenty-first birthday, my older brother was in a motorcycle accident that left him paralyzed. The first weeks after his accident were touch-and-go.

My precious mama wanted all of her friends around. My dad wanted them all to go away. My oldest brother wanted to be in my brother's room in the center of all of the information and I hid in a stairwell, holding my breath.

While we were all in different places in how we experienced our grief, we were all right in how we experienced our grief. We may have done so differently but we did it in ways that were true and authentic to each of us.

You and your partner are both experiencing your own emotions, but doing so very differently.

However you may be experiencing this season, doing so in a constructive manner is appropriate. Just make sure that you are sharing it with your partner and creating space for them to be emotionally present with you, too.

Have times that you set aside to discuss your emotions and pain. Maybe you need a set meeting time or just to allow the moments to be authentic. However you do it, make sure that you allow yourselves the time to process together.

Take Timeouts

While we talk about the importance of emotional intimacy in a relationship, we also need to consider the importance of taking timeouts.

What would it feel like to go on a date with your partner and not talk about infertility? Imagine the beauty of not discussing cycle days, Gonal F injections, who offended you with their ignorant remarks, the minefields of pregnancy announcements on social media, or trying to agree on who we should tell about your pain.

It truly is exhausting, isn't it?

Let me remind you that there is so much more to your relationship than infertility. If we were to look at a pie chart of who you and your partner are, just a sliver of that pie would be infertility. It does feel like much more, I do realize.

What are your hobbies? What did you love discussing when you were falling in love? What dreams did you share? What were your inspirations? What brought out your creative side? Who or what did you cheer for?

On occasion, give yourself permission to spend time on all of the other aspects of who you and your partner are, while putting all of your fertility strife on the shelf. Go on a date and don't touch it. Have some deep belly laughs together. High-five each other after you bowl a strike. Live like it was the good-old-days before infertility hijacked your happiness.

There is time to discuss infertility. Find a time for it together. But, also find time to shelf it. It is important for any relationship that you find the balance of both business and non-business and in this case, dealing with the reality of infertility versus the other parts of your relationship.

Self-care

While we identify the lengths that we must go to be on Team Marriage inside of a relationship, I would be remiss if we didn't discuss the importance of individual self-care.

In order to truly thrive, we also need to identify what helps you come alive individually.

Perhaps it is a bubble bath, a phone call with a dear friend, a match on the sand volleyball court, a wine night with the girls, or a walk alone in the wilderness. Whatever it is that makes you take the deepest of breaths or find the truest nature of your soul, do that. What makes one come alive will not be all the ingredients for another friend to find herself.

Whatever it is for you, be all there. Tap completely into it. Make it a complete priority. Make yourself a priority.

Ideally, what comes after infertility is pregnancy and then the season of postpartum and then parenthood. The following seasons, even if it includes childlessness, are not good times to be focusing our starting your self-care regiment. Now is the time to start any new practices.

Looking Back

Life always ends for me in a hospice bed. I know this just took a really morbid turn, but go with me here.

When I picture the end of my days, I picture myself in a bed with my family all circled around my bed. We're reminiscing because I'm a reminiscer.

In those moments, I want to be able to confidently say that I lived well. In the highs and the lows, I want to recall how we grew out of it. I want to look back on my life and say that even on the most difficult of days, I dug deep, found my strength, and persevered. I want to say that I loved well and with intention. I don't want to look back on my life and recall the pockets of life that I missed out on.

I believe this so strongly because there was a pocket of my life that I let control me. Yes, my husband and I can say that we grew out of the experience, but the days were really long and hard.

I look back over those years and what I remember is the young woman hiding in bed because the outside world was fertile and I wasn't. I remember the tears that fell like rain as I sat in one of the deepest valleys of my life. I remember avoiding instead of living. I remember the seething anger, the calloused interactions, and jealous rage. Those are not a good color on anyone.

The passion behind my work as a Reproductive Therapist is because I want you to live well in the wait. I want your hindsight to give you the greatest gift of resiliency, overcoming, and courage.

I want you to look back and say, "I lived well. I thrived."

What changes do you need to make so that you can live more intentionally now?

What do you and your partner need to do to be on Team Marriage again? What do you need to do to take care of yourself?

What do you need to do so when your story ends, you can say: "I lived well. I thrived."

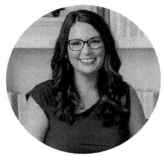

Cathie Quillet
Marriage & Family Therapist
www.nashvillereproductivetherapy.com
www.thequilletinstitute.com

Cathie Quillet is a Licensed Marriage and Family Therapist and owner of Nashville Reproductive Therapy in her hometown of Nashville, TN. Additionally, Cathie is a Fertility Coach, Published Author, Public Speaker & barren Mom who specializes in infertility and pregnancy loss, along with the treatment of those in the seasons of pregnancy, postpartum and adoption.

Cathie is passionate about serving women all over the world, which is why she founded The Quillet Institute. A passion project offering coaching, comfort and an actual pathway for women and their partners to work through emotional struggles that comes with infertility. (www.thequilletinstitute.com)

Cathie is a member of Resolve and is a trained member of the American Society of Reproductive Medicine. Additionally, Cathie is the Counseling Advisor for Waiting in Hope.

Cathie is the author of the books Not Pregnant: A Companion for the Emotional Journey of Infertility, No Matter What Happens and the Peace (In)Fertility Workbook, which is a companion to her online video program.

Learning to Breathe in a Vacuum

By Dr. Dan Schaefer

I can't recall a time when I heard a young married couple morbidly predict that they would probably have great difficulty getting pregnant. Unless there is a known prohibitive medical condition at the outset, or they are a card-carrying member of the Pessimist's Society, most couples who want children are relatively optimistic about getting pregnant and delivering a healthy baby. And rightly so. So, when pregnancy does not occur right away (or at all), or repeated miscarriages ensue, most couples are largely unprepared for the uncertain road ahead of them. This chapter is written to help those couples who are traveling along the unpredictable road of infertility to stay connected to both each other and their friends and family.

Numbers

Many mental health practitioners hate numbers. I actually like them. I taught a research course for graduate students for almost a decade. It felt like a campaign to sell them on a political candidate that they hated, or about whom they had heard terrible things...second hand. Hopefully, some of them learned something, or at least did not projectile vomit when they heard the word "STA-TIS-TICS."

Outside the classroom, most couples use numbers and statistics when they are balancing their checkbook, predicting the weather, or calculating a tip after a good meal. However, should they experience a significant delay in becoming pregnant, and the months of anticipation slowly turn from disappointment to long seasons of heartache, the math-phobic suddenly become math majors: "What do you mean, three out of ten? What are our chances of getting pregnant "on our own?" "What is the phone number of the local OB-GYN fertility magician? What is his/her success rate? How long will this take? How much does it cost? Should we increase our chances by going to a bigger, out-of-town medical center?"

If you bought this book, you already know more about fertility rates than you want to, so I won't waste any space with probabilities. You already know you are in a painful minority.

Life in A Vacuum

Mr. Carr was my socially awkward 7th grade science teacher in his first year of teaching. He did an experiment that I still remember. He started with a palm-sized alarm clock with a little hammer that alternately struck two little brass bells. He would wind up the alarm clock, and let it ring. As it was still ringing, he would then quickly cover the clock with a bell jar, melt wax around the base, and turn on a pump that sucked all the air out of the jar. Very quickly the bell went silent as we watched, wide-eyed and open-mouthed, as the little hammer continued to pound away. The lesson learned was that sound waves need air to travel. But what I also remember from Mr. Carr's class that day was the sound of air rushing back into the jar the second he broke the paraffin seal.

Nature hates a vacuum.

People also hate a vacuum.

Suppose you are traveling on the interstate and hear a new whirring sound. You get curious and try to make sense of it. You either comfort yourself with some useful fiction (the car is fine; it's the surface of the road) or pull over and get to the bottom of it. In most cases, our natural curiosity and/or distaste for the vacuum motivates us to fill the void. However, there are some cases when that option is either impossible or completely out of our control.

Infertility is one of those cases.

Infertility is a painful, information-poor environment; a hated vacuum where we can easily fall prey to a universal human tendency: in the absence of information, we tend to assume the worst. As time rolls on, infertile couples may find themselves assuming the worst in three dimensions: the future, our partner, and ourselves.

It is rather common to be reserved, worried or even pessimistic about one's future; about finding a good job, being happily married, or experiencing good health. Infertile couples walk this same tight rope between a hopeful future and the possibility of never having biological children of their own as they invest and wait. While not uncommon, this particular wait is unusually intense.

Evil Twins: Shame and Blame

The infertility waiting room is no place for the weak. It is also no place for isolation. For there is no better environment than isolation for two brutal realities to emerge and take over: blame and shame. Blame and shame can run quietly in the background, filling our vacuum with near-savage thoughts about your partner and yourself that can leak into conversations and emotional reactions in subtle and surprising ways.

As the months turn into years, and the bank account is being drained, and most of your friends are having multiple children, more troubling questions emerge: Why is this happening? What did we do wrong? Are we being punished? Does God hate us? Why are all these freaking teenagers getting knocked up? Whose fault is this anyhow? Is what they say about tighty whities actually true? Will we ever have spontaneous sex again? Are my best sperm still sticking to some sheets in my bachelor's pad? The list of possible questions could go on, but you get the idea. Since most of the answers to these questions are never found, and nature hates a vacuum, it is inevitable that the misery crescendos with the most devastating question that any infertile couple can ask themselves: "What is wrong with me/you/us?"

There is an old adage, "Under stress, we tend to regress."

In other words, we start thinking like younger versions of ourselves, like children. Developmental literature tells us that it is easier to take the blame for something, even if it is hardly plausible than it is to live with a mystery unsolved. A little four-year-old girl loses her dad to a heart attack as he was reading her a book as she sat on his lap. For years, on the edge of her consciousness, she entertained the thought that she had killed her father. Not only would any normal friend or parent ever agree with that logic, but they would do their best to tenderly set her thinking straight. Why? Because grownups have a bit of an advantage over four-year-olds...in most cases. Unlike four-year-olds, adults usually can articulate these internal dialogues with good friends, family, or a therapist, who can gently bring perspective to that quiet brutality. But this brutality can be strongly associated with a deeply troubling and painful human emotion: shame.

Shame

In the past few decades, social psychology has taught us that the human experience of shame is associated with nothing helpful. Research has indicated that it is correlated with depression, anger, anxiety, excessive alcohol consumption, and social withdrawal. I am convinced that this mostly hidden feeling is often rearing its ugly head in the quiet thoughts of both men and women who have embarked on the infertility journey. At the root of shame-filled feelings is a pernicious idea: "There is something deeply flawed within me. I am defective" As these thoughts build, they can compete with actual truth. I cannot emphasize how deep-seated and devastating this "master emotion" can be. Left unaddressed, most humans will propel themselves into emotional seclusion; the exact state that will perpetuate and extend the effects of shame.

The remedy is to look carefully at the rebuilding of interpersonal bridges, which we will discuss in the next section. I am not sure that this extremely painful emotion can be remedied on one's own. In fact, it may be impossible.

Blame

The third leg of this three-legged stool is blame. Driven again by the aversion of the vacuum, we assume the worst, this time about our partner. Whether the blame is spoken or not, in isolation one could begin weaving a logical but unscientific story of how past attitudes or behaviors of your partner somehow led to current infertility. This fiction may be a temporary balm for shame, but will no doubt be a corrosive element in your bond with your partner.

Being A Friend To Yourself and Your Partner

Harriet Learner, a psychologist whose career addressed the complexities of domestic violence stated, "If you can do only one thing for a woman who is trapped in an abusive relationship, get her out of isolation." I can't think of a more applicable strategy for the pain of infertility. And it should start with your spouse. I have been seeing couples in therapy for over three decades, some of whom were smart enough to engage in premarital counseling. I have marveled at the diversity of abilities to engage in meaningful and/or conflictual dialogue. These abilities are often replications of how we were raised. Many couples seeking infertility services are in the early stages of marriage; maybe even the "honeymoon stage." Either way, if this is the first big challenge in the relationship, having the skills to process these emotional complexities is crucial.

These are several great tools to help couples stay connected through conflict, Harville Hendrix's Getting the Love You Want is a highly recommended resource whose title is self-explanatory. Bottom line: I think you can assume that your partner has thoughts that he/she does not want to talk about, as do you. And if other concerns are consuming a lot of your attention, the bigger issues, such as fears of being deeply flawed, may be ignored altogether.

If I can get couples to spend time together, I encourage them to regularly sit with their partner on a couch facing each other for half an hour. One talks and the other listens; the latter periodically summarizing what the speaker says and feels, without ever interjecting their reactions or opinions. At the 15 minute mark, reverse roles. If the complexity of the infertility increases, many couples increase the length or the frequency of these "mirroring" sessions. There may be no more effective way for couples to dredge up all that is going on inside them and connect deeply with their partner (and it is cheaper than professional therapy). Since shame seems to drive us into isolation as it spreads like black mold in our basement, breaking out of that silence is the essence of healing the shame or blame that is lodged deep within us.

Teaching Others How to Be Your Friend

I shared an office years ago with a friend and colleague who had the following phrase framed: "I teach people how I want to be treated." I originally thought this was too cutesy and kind of stupid. A month later I was routinely pointing to that sign during my sessions.

Almost every couple I talk to who has struggled with infertility has a story or two about hurtful things that people say to them about their dilemma. The great irony is that while the comments feel mean-spirited, they were typically trying to help! These well-meaning comments may come out of ignorance, or carelessness, or their discomfort with suffering. Regardless, friends need to be taught how you want to be treated.

The Old Testament book about Job is a story about a wealthy, decent, God-following man who encounters massive losses of family, possessions, and even personal health, for no discernable reason whatsoever. As you could imagine, he was a wreck; grieving, alone, and scraping the scabs on his body with broken shards of pottery. When his three friends first encounter him, they could not even recognize him.

When they finally did, they wept loudly, and as was the custom, tore their clothing and threw dust on their heads to express their support. Their initial beautiful attempt to accompany their friend was soon replaced by a spectacular disaster in my eyes and has massive implications for all grieving infertile couples.

Their support began well: "Then they sat on the ground with him for seven days and seven nights. No one said a word to him, because they saw how great his suffering was." (Job 2:13). But then they opened their mouths and neutralized all the kindness and wisdom they had first displayed.

If in the middle of the infertility vacuum you have the company of close friends and family who can tolerate mystery and ambiguity, and who understand how healing their "non-explaining" presence is, you have found a treasure.

If you are lucky you won't have to explain this to everyone. Some, particularly other couples who have struggled with infertility, already get this. For those who don't, I have two ideas. First, catch them doing it right. If you open up to friends or family, and they simply sit with you like Job's friends, remind them repeatedly how much you appreciate their attentive company. And remember, this is not a passive activity. Talk to any therapist who comes home exhausted after sitting in a comfortable chair all day. Listening to suffering is hard work. Secondly, when the vacuum is filled with ideas from your friends who become restless and begin trying to "help" but instead wound you, speak up. "Jane, I have no doubt that you are trying to be helpful, but your words are becoming wounding to me." "Sue, your optimism about our infertility is well-intended, but it is starting to drive a wedge between us." "Fred, your humor about sperm counts is no longer funny to me." "Jack, we may well decide to adopt a child, but if that happens, it does not make our infertility any less painful."

Our Story

My wife and I used to go to church with a couple in their late 30's who had no children, even though they married early and had never used birth control. Anne was generally in good health, so when she developed a headache and chills in her late 30's, she saw her family doctor who happened to be a member of their church. When their physician could find nothing wrong and asked, "Is there any chance that you are pregnant?" they both laughed out loud. Ten minutes later, they found out they were pregnant. It gets even better: two years later they gave birth to their second healthy little girl.

Around this same time, my wife Shelly and I were in the middle of our second expensive round of IVF; shots in her thigh, travel out of state and handing my little cup of Olympic swimmers to a nurse I will never recognize (because I was looking at my shoes at the handoff before dashing down the hospital corridor).

We were hopeful. Our first round was grueling and culminated in a hospitalization. This second time seemed different. We had done all our homework, read all the books, and had the support of our friends and family. I was at a professional convention when I got the news that Shelly had miscarried again. We knew that the havoc our attempts left on Shelly's body and spirit had to come to an end. I left the conference early and booked the first flight back home the next morning.

Overall, our friends were terrific. It makes me cringe to think of how many infertile couples go through similar ordeals but without the connection and support of friends and family. They seemed to know that we needed time with them; not answers or (worse) EXPLANATIONS!! Those two latter things are excruciating; like getting too much sun at the beach the first day, then being forced out into that sun the next day without an umbrella or sunscreen.

Parting Shot

Couples who have not or cannot get pregnant need a lot of things. The one thing they do NOT need is an explanation of any sort (carelessly or meticulously reasoned) as to WHY this is happening to them. Any explanation, even if it is asked for, is like giving your infertile friends a drug that is not only ineffective but also has long term, massive side-effects; while providing great "clarity/comfort" only to the explainer. The best way friends and family can help is by not letting you get away with treating yourself like an enemy or descending into the abyss of self-name-calling and shame.

In conclusion, I return to Mr. Carr and his bell jar. Nature and people hate a vacuum; so much so that we will invent all sorts of "useful fictions" to avoid the distress of not knowing answers. If you are on this infertility journey, guard your heart; never say anything to yourself that you would never say to an infertile friend. Teach your friends that there are no good explanations for why this is happening to you. Any suggestions they could offer are likely light-years behind what you have already considered. Any explanation they could offer would be redundant, and likely wrong and hurtful. Instead, remind them how their friendship is to you, and the richness of having them just sit with you as you and your partner maneuver through this heartache. Catch them doing it right and relieve them of having to make sense of it all. And when in doubt, be gentle with yourself and your partner. This journey will not be in vain.

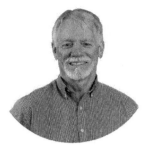

Dr. Dan Schaefer
Licensed Psychologist
www.pprweb.net

Dan Schaefer, Ph.D. is a psychologist and director of Person to Person Resources, Inc., a private mental health practice in Toledo, Ohio. He works with adolescents and adults, occasionally seeing younger children as a part of family therapy. He has worked extensively with high conflict couples, as well as having run groups for 10 years for men arrested for domestic violence. Other areas if specialization include shame and guilt issues, pornography addiction, recovery from extramarital affairs, and EMDR.

Stress Reduction Options to Get You Through Treatment

By Lisa Schuman

It all started with my family building journey. Before my husband and I married, we decided to consult with my gynecologist. My mother had a miscarriage before having me, and her doctor suggested she take a medication called diethylstilbestrol (DES), which was given to women in the 1960's to help prevent miscarriages. These women, born between 1938 and 1971, were at risk for many reproductive difficulties including a rare form of cancer. Fortunately, I did not develop cancer, but I did have reproductive problems. My doctor thought I was fine, so I wasn't worried until our fertility doctor told me I had an "infantile uterus."

I also had irregular periods, so I took fertility medication and underwent surgery to clear my uterus of any scar tissue or blockages and began fertility treatment. After multiple rounds of IUI and IVF and two losses, we were back at ground zero.

So, we did what most desperate people would do. We tried everything. When every medical procedure that was available at the time didn't work, we drank smelly concoctions from an herbalist in a five-story walkup in Chinatown. I had acupuncture, I visualized and didn't visualize, I meditated and prayed and then didn't. I tried several different diets, took supplements, tried new exercises, and religious rituals. Our neighbors complained because the concoction I was cooking every day with turtle nails and horse whiskers (not really, but I'm sure it was something like that) was so foul, you could smell it down the hallway in my apartment building. Imagine what that tasted like!

We turned to surrogacy, and at the time, surrogacy was not as common on the East Coast as it is now. There were no boilerplate contracts and our surrogate, who we wined and dined, periodically sent our attorney requests for more money, even after our contract was finalized. We were worried she would continue this through the pregnancy and we would feel held hostage.

We were exhausted and depressed. Our moods were down, we had very little energy, and my self-esteem was in the toilet.

I felt terrible about my body. I always dreamt of being pregnant. I used to tell my girlfriends that I wanted a huge belly and I would love every minute of it. I had no attachment to my genetics, but I wanted to experience pregnancy. I played with dolls as a child and spent my young adult life trying not to get pregnant. I assumed my plan for a big and joyful pregnancy was inevitable. Why not? This was my plan and isn't that the way things work? When you want something, you make a plan, work hard, and get it. Right?

It was also my husband's plan. I'll never forget the day we learned I was pregnant. He said, "I have never been so happy." Every loss and disappointment after that felt so much worse because I remembered those words and felt so sad for him too.

If you have been up and down on the fertility roller coaster, you know that the pain you feel in your heart may be exacerbated by the pain you feel in your wallet. We had very little insurance coverage for treatment and spent so much money that we had no money left for pleasurable activities. As a young couple, we had hoped to put money away for retirement and also enjoy our lives together, but there was little joy. I don't need to get into the drudgery, intrusive nature, and exhausting and consuming experience of fertility treatment. So much has been written about that already, and if you have been down that road, you completely understand. For some, that process is relatively quick, and for others, it is long and fraught with difficulties. We were in the second camp.

When I came to the place where I wanted the pain to end and my desire to become pregnant was overshadowed by the desire to parent, we turned to adoption. My husband wanted to keep trying. Our new marriage was in turmoil. We were both in individual therapy and couple's therapy. Finally, we mended our relationship and decided to adopt. The world of fertility treatment had taught us a new language and how to navigate a world we didn't want to be a part of. It was so difficult to accept every new phase of treatment and even harder to experience. We were sad and exhausted... and...we were starting over.

There were many ups and downs on the adoption road as well, and we made many mistakes along the way. We finally found the right people and learned the shortcuts. Enduring these experiences made me determined to find an easier path to parenthood for my patients. I vowed to help prevent others from making the same or similar mistakes and enduring unnecessary stress. The world of reproductive medicine is so different now. Some options weren't available when I was trying, and much more research exists on stress and managing the difficulties of fertility treatment.

Over the more than two decades as a family building therapist, I have had the privilege to lecture across the country, teach other professionals, and advocate for families-to-be. I have won awards for my research from the American Society for Reproductive Medicine and the Pacific Coast Reproductive Society. I am Director of Mental Health Services for Reproductive Medicine Associates of Connecticut and Gay Parents to Be, and Founder and Director for the Center for Family Building. I enjoy my work and the ever-changing landscape of reproductive medicine. However, my greatest joy is helping people achieve their dreams of building their families. And I have been fortunate to have helped thousands of people.

The internet is full of contradicting and confusing information. At the Center for Family Building, we can cut through the noise and provide people with the information they need to navigate treatment effectively and the tools they need to manage their stress and relationships while they are on their path to parenthood. One person may feel their family is full with one child, and another may feel that unless they have three children, their family is not complete. An ideal situation for some may be to use a friend or sibling as a donor and for others that would be a total disaster. Everyone deserves to feel fulfilled and whole in attaining their dreams to build their unique family structure.

For many, having a baby can take time. Success rates have increased dramatically over the past two decades, and donor conception and surrogacy are easier and more effective than ever. But the process of building your family with reproductive medicine needs to be done correctly.

Without the right guidance, it is easy to choose the wrong agency or donor. For example, it is important to know that all donors and surrogates should have proper screening, including an evaluation by a trained mental health professional and psychological testing (the PAI and MMPI are the most widely-respected tests at the time of this writing). It is also important for everyone using third-party reproduction (donor eggs, donor sperm, or surrogacy) to consider issues such as disclosure and genetics carefully. Also, it is essential to choose a good clinic and think ahead about your long-term goals before making decisions. Resolving these issues can help people have the families they desire in less time, and with less chance of regret.

Get sound, professional guidance from professionals who have been working in reproductive medicine for a long time and are actively involved with the American Society for Reproductive Medicine. If you were having heart surgery, wouldn't you want to see a surgeon who has performed hundreds of the same surgeries and is affiliated with the most prominent related medical association? Why would you take your family building journey any less seriously?

Now that you have the right mindset to proactively get the help you need, let's review some ways of managing your emotions while you go through treatment. Research has shown that women undergoing fertility treatment can experience similar levels of depression as chemotherapy patients. It may be hard to imagine that this is true, but if you have been through treatment, you may be all too familiar with feelings of anxiety or depression. Perhaps your friends and family members don't understand how difficult treatment can be, but as one of my patients aptly said, "it can take the stuffing out of you."

There are many reasons why treatment is challenging, but perhaps the most common reaction when undergoing fertility treatment is feeling the effects of the "fight or flight response."

Herbert Benson, MD, was perhaps the first researcher in the U.S. who wrote about the idea of practicing relaxation techniques to bring our heart rate and blood pressure to a healthy state.

Believe it or not, the "fight or flight response" is similar for all animals. When a rabbit feels that a predator is near, the hair goes up on the back of his neck, his heart starts racing, and his pupils dilate. He is ready to flee or fight. Nature has given us this gift for survival, but once the threat has passed, we can relax. The problem is that with fertility treatment, this feeling is triggered over and over, creating tension and a build-up of cortisol (the stress hormone) in our systems. An abundance of cortisol is not good for your mood or your health.

This chapter will outline three ways to manage the stress of fertility treatment. For more tools or to receive guidance from our professionally-trained therapists, contact us at www.familybuilding.net. But before we talk about techniques, you must let go of regrets and understand that you are entitled to have the family of your dreams.

Empower Yourself

Many people feel they are undeserving. Some people tell me it is "not right" to be a single parent or that adoption is "better" because there are so many children who need "saving" in the world. The truth is that thousands of people hope to adopt a healthy baby each year, so there is no shortage of people to adopt those children. The children who need "saving" are the children in the foster care system who have emotional or intellectual difficulties. Those children truly need good homes, but if you are not prepared to take on the responsibility of caring for a child with difficulties, you should not do it.

Some people feel that God or nature does not want them to have a child and their infertility is evidence of this fact. Yet those same people are willing to be immunized against diseases, attend physical therapy appointments to recover from minor injuries, and wear braces to correct crooked teeth. However, when it comes to building a family, many people are reluctant to feel proud and entitled to have the family they desire. If this is you, I urge you to think about this and make a clear decision to go after the family of your dreams with strength and determination

Mindset

It's been said that our mind creates the world we live in. A positive mindset has been credited for the success of business people, athletes, and heads of state. Changing your mindset can change your life long-term, and short-term it can bring about a happier and more relaxed state. I have chosen a few of my favorite stress reduction techniques to help you change your mindset.

The goal is not to snap your fingers and feel differently about everything. The goal is to move to a better feeling state. There is a place for sadness and grief, but it is also helpful not to stay in that place. Our bodies will always look for problems. It is natural to focus on problems and to get stuck ruminating over the problems of the past or worries about the future. Allowing yourself to have your feelings and then to attempt to move, even a little, to a better place is the goal. It is a helpful way to care for yourself and your children. So, consider these strategies as tools for you and your future family.

The following example may help you bring this idea into better focus. Your child is getting dressed for school and he trips and falls in the kitchen. His skinned knee is bleeding and he looks at you with tears running down his face. Your child is upset about his knee, feels frightened at the sight of his injury, and decides the that worst thing in the world has just happened.

Although you console him, he says he can't go to school. Do you let him stay home? No. You clean the wound, patch it up with a Band-Aid, and give him a big hug. Then you tell him he will be fine and get him ready for school. You neither ignore his feelings and simply push him to go to school nor spend hours upset with him while letting him stay home.

He needs time for his feelings but also needs to feel empowered and learn that he can overcome a small injury. This experience will help him build confidence and also teach him that all of his feelings are valuable. Why treat yourself any differently?

The stress reduction strategies described in this chapter are organized into three categories. 1. Decreasing negative emotions. 2. Increasing positive emotions. 3. Managing overwhelm (or feeling out of control). Many people use the first, decreasing negative emotions, most. When negative feelings emerge, it is often reflexive to try to "get rid" of the feelings that are causing discomfort. However, using tools to increase positive feelings and to manage feelings of "out of control" or overwhelm are also very helpful. It is best if you use some tips from each category.

Your background, temperament, and where you are in your life right now will determine the mix that works best for you. This list serves as an example of these categories, but it is not exhaustive. Feel free to add your tips to the categories and continue to mix and match the strategies until you find the right balance.

As treatment evolves, your symptoms may change. This may necessitate returning to this list to add new or different strategies to your toolbox. Managing your emotions is more like eating from a buffet than ordering an entrée from a menu. No one strategy works for everyone, and ideally, you will have a variety of strategies that you can use at different times for different moods.

Decreasing Negative Emotions

- *Be mindful of your body.* The internet is full of companies offering free exercise, stretching, dance classes, Pilates, yoga classes, and more. There are many options on social media for "dance parties" and exercise instruction. If you are tired of looking at your computer, don't be afraid to play a song, dance around the house, and sing out loud. It's almost impossible to feel down while dancing to your favorite song.

When your posture is poor, you tend to feel worse. Think about how you stand or sit when you are feeling upset vs. feeling happy. This is a "fake it 'til you make it strategy" and is supported by research. So, sit up straight, even when you don't feel like it. A small adjustment in posture can change your attitude.

- *Take care of your mind.* During times of crisis, your mind may be in overdrive. The best way to quiet the mind is meditation. It is important not to dismiss meditation out of hand.

There are many types of meditation and many meditation apps and YouTube videos that are free or low cost. Try a few before you decide you don't like it.

Therapy can be extremely useful too. The Mental Health Professional Group of the American Society for Reproductive Medicine is a great resource. Try a few different therapists before you commit. I often say that people spend more time choosing a pair of shoes they like than a therapist with whom they will truly connect. Lastly, stress reduction strategies such as tapping have helped many in times of crisis. A variety of these strategies are also easily accessible on YouTube.

Yoga has been called moving meditation. If you have trouble sitting still, yoga may be a way for you to quiet your mind while still moving your body. Just like meditation, yoga is called a practice because the more you do it, the better the effect. It is not natural to be "good at it" right away but with regular practice (just like most things in life) many have experienced tremendous benefits.

- *Go on a Google diet.* While keeping up with the latest technologies may feel important, the stress that naturally develops from ingesting all of the conflicting information and fear can have a significant effect on your psyche. Learn what you need to know, find the right doctor, and follow their guidance. Since negative messages can be so disruptive to your mood, if you must indulge, it is best not to do so before you go to bed or if you are feeling an increased level of stress.
- *Take turns.* If you are in a partnership and have children at home, it is extremely important to give each other time to "take breaks" from the children and housework. This may mean going to bed earlier so you can get up earlier when the house is quiet, or finding separate activities to do with the children.
- *Follow the twenty-minute rule.* If conversations about fertility treatment are dominating your life, plan to speak about it for only twenty minutes a day. If you or your partner have a fertility-related thought, write it down and save it for the next day.

Increase Positive Emotions

- *Get outside.* Moving your body is important, but it is also helpful to take a walk outside when possible. Feeling the sun or wind on your face and smelling the scents outside your home activates your senses and can have a positive effect on your well-being.
- *Give.* When you give to others, you give to yourself. After performing an act of kindness, you may notice that you feel more joy and inner peace. There are many opportunities online to sew masks, send pictures of homemade cards to homebound people, donate, or take a class to be certified to offer support on a hotline.
- *Laugh.* Even if you are feeling down, a funny movie, book or video can help pull you out of your slump. There are many accounts of people finding healing through laughter.
- *Connect.* Make time to connect with people inside and outside of your household. Religious organizations, community centers, and

other groups have created online platforms for connecting as well. Play board games or puzzles or take hikes together. Even if you feel that you are only distracted 20% of the time, that means 80% of the time you were focused on your journey and that is better than 100%.

- *Think about what you can enjoy rather than what you cannot enjoy.* Our bodies are programmed to look for problems. You can counteract this reflex by remembering your goal is to get through treatment as pleasurably as possible. Then focus on things you can do rather than things you cannot do.
- *Practice gratitude.* The saying, "gratitude will change your attitude" may seem hokey, but it works. Research backs it up. You can start by saying, writing, and thinking about 3-5 things you are grateful for each day. Even if life is unbelievably challenging, finding anything you can feel grateful for, even if it is just that you are breathing, can elevate your mood.

Managing Overwhelm (Or Feeling Out of Control)

- *Engage in productive and pleasurable activities.* This could mean reorganizing your living room, taking an online drawing class, or learning how to knit. Not knowing what will happen next, waiting for test results, or worrying about getting disappointing news can leave you feeling out of control and dysregulated. When you put your energy into an activity that is pleasurable and productive, not only do you have a pleasurable distraction, but seeing a result from your efforts can feel very stabilizing.
- *Stay on a schedule.* Going to bed and waking at the same time each day is beneficial for your health and emotional well-being. When you are stressed, it can feel tempting to stay up late or "sleep in." Maintaining a schedule can help you sleep better at night; help you feel productive and keep your household in sync.

It's been said that we can't control what happens to us, but we can control how we react. We have control over our choices of doctors, donors, agencies, timing, and the treatments we choose, but there is so much that is not within our control. This fact can feel maddening. The natural response many people have when they intensely want something and it is not working is to focus more and try harder. While this strategy works in many areas of life, it does not work in fertility treatment.

In fact, focusing more on treatment will only cause more frustration and cause the experience of treatment to slow down, and no one wants that. No one wants to relish every exam and blood draw. It would be ideal if you could start treatment, go to sleep, and wake up pregnant. Unfortunately, we can't make that happen, but using the strategies outlined in this chapter will not only reduce your level of stress but can help treatment seem like it is moving more quickly.

Further, research shows that even when treatment is affordable, patients stop trying because it is so stressful. Don't let stress stop you from reaching your goals. With a little practice and focus on managing your stress, you are more likely to be able to improve your mood so you can better tolerate treatment and achieve the family you desire.

And feel free to reach out to us anytime at www.familybuilding.net. Our goal is to help you have an easier journey to parenthood.

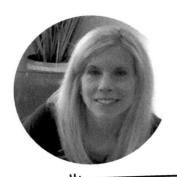

Lisa Schuman
Licensed Clinical Social Worker
www.familybuilding.net

Lisa Schuman, LCSW, is a leading expert in family building and has helped people around globe build the families of their dreams.

She has lectured extensively and has written numerous articles on a variety of family building subjects including LGBTQ, and single parent family building. Ms. Schuman also runs workshops and offers counseling for parents and children who have formed their families through sperm and egg donation or adoption.

She has been working as a licensed therapist for more than two decades and is currently the Director of Mental Health Services for Reproductive Medicine Associates of Connecticut and Gay Parents to Be. She is a consultant for schools and corporations and has worked with groups such as Memorial Sloane Kettering, The Gay and Lesbian Community Center, The Family Equality Council and Single Mothers by Choice.

Lisa, who lives in New York with her husband and three children, has personally experienced almost every facet of family building including fertility treatment, surgeries, alternative therapies, surrogacy and adoption and has lived through the struggles raising mainstream and special needs children. This has given her special insight into the trials, tribulations and joys of the families she counsels. Says Schuman, "I can talk the talk but I have also walked the walk."

Five Things I learned From Adoption After Infertility

By Dr. Mark Trolice

Creating a family is considered by many the foundation of our existence and often defines our entry to adulthood. Despite over 40 years of advances in assisted reproductive technologies, infertility remains a devastating diagnosis and, often, a costly, demanding, uncertain journey toward the goal of a healthy baby. Once labeled, infertility patients may feel overwhelmed, anxious, depressed, isolated, and "broken", to name only a few symptoms.

For those with infertility, the notion of successful reproduction becomes a foreign concept that permeates the minds of all those struggling. While having a child and growing a family are common goals among us, the inability to reproduce has a self-imposed negative value. Couples, particularly women, label themselves as "inadequate" and even "failures" as a consequence of not being able to have a child.

Cultural perspectives may also increase the challenge of infertility because both women and men can be stigmatized. In Africa, the true meaning of marriage is defined as being only fulfilled if the couple is able to successfully have a child. (Hum Reprod 2004;19:960-7). Third-party reproduction and adoption in India are pursued secretly to avoid the visible admission of infertility. (Soc Sci Med 2003;56:1867-80)

Managing infertility, patients can endure a significant physical, financial, and emotional investment. The advanced reproductive technology of in vitro fertilization (IVF) involves the woman receive daily injections of hormones and undergo an egg retrieval that is costly and often not covered by insurance. A treatment cycle is often described as an "emotional roller coaster" due to the myriad effects of hormonal medications combined with the stress of the unknown outcome. The psychological symptoms associated with infertility, such as anxiety and depression, are similar to those associated with other serious medical conditions such as cancer and cardiac rehabilitation. (J Psychosom Obstet Gynaecol 1993;14 Suppl:45-52)

For many, the trauma of receiving this diagnosis often equals the realization of needing treatment. Unfortunately, patients have shared with me that acquiescing to therapy crushes the dream of the unjust mindset that conception should be natural, or it was "not meant to be." Seemingly, no other field of medicine demonstrates the ambivalence of infertility patients toward treatment.

Along every infertility patient's journey, the questions that haunt both waking hours and dreams, "was I meant to have a child?" In over 20 years of caring for infertility patients, I consider this question, above all others, as the most unfair and defeating. From an evolutionary perspective, every adult was meant to have a child. From a social perspective, one can argue, all caring, mature, financially stable, and responsible people are meant and deserve to have a child. Yet, as infertility prolongs, patients begin to, unjustly, contemplate their worthiness. Alas, an additional unnecessary burden on this devastated population.

Nevertheless, fertility and infertility (with exceptions) are endowed by nature. The biological ability to conceive and bear a child should not be a gauge whereby one is judged as having merit. Rather, one should be measured by their virtue. To quote author Leo Buscaglia, "Your talent is God's gift to you. What you do with it is your gift back to God." (Buscaglia, L. F., & Short, S. (1982). Living, loving & learning. Thorofare, N.J: C.B. Slack.)

How do I know all this? After 20 years of treating infertility patients and 10 years of personally enduring infertility, I have gained a unique perspective on the psychological and emotional turmoil the disease produces. And so, it is through my experience of resolving infertility and adopting five angels that I provide insight into alternative methods of family building. The knowledge I have gained allows me to compare the joy and fulfillment of adoption to the gratification of natural conception.

First

As a stubborn Italian from the New York metro area in Northern New Jersey, I was determined to have biological children. Adoption was as foreign to me as, well, Southern New Jersey – we just didn't go there. After all, we were only trying for several years, so what's a few more? The simple answer: a horrendous emotional toll.

Admittedly, I was embarrassed. No one in my family ever adopted a child. Would they treat my child differently from other biologically related children? Would cousins play with my child? Would my wife and I still feel self-imposed ostracism? These questions suffocated my mind and prolonged our decision because of "analysis-paralysis," my preferred term for over-thinking to the point of mindful entrapment.

Our struggle with infertility influenced time to seemingly stand still and pass rapidly, simultaneously. Three years became five then seven and finally 10. During our decade of infertility, we endured surgery, multiple

IUI (intrauterine insemination) cycles, multiple IVF (in vitro fertilization) cycles resulting in miscarriage, ectopic pregnancy, ovarian hyperstimulation syndrome, and multiple negative pregnancy tests. One other tragic outcome, social withdrawal - from family, friends, and, sadly, each other but fortunately only temporarily. The strain on a couple's relationship from infertility is the proverbial "elephant in the room," i.e., it's always there yet one only rarely, if ever, acknowledges.

Just as one's infertility treatment evolves, so did my perspective on the meaning of family. My loving wife broached the subject of adoption somewhere between years 5-7 of our quest. Following our last unsuccessful IVF cycle, the number to which I avoid committing memory, I shared my support to build our family through the miracle of adoption.

What a magnanimous gesture by a birth giver. She clearly had the right to options, yet she chose to provide the baby with a life to which she was not capable. On the receiving end, there are the intended parents who await, with open arms, a non-biological child to, whole-heartedly, nurture, and love. Truly, a miraculous process and one for which I will remain grateful for the rest of my life.

Second

When young, we are often guided toward having a family of our own, i.e. biologically. What we rarely learn is the interruption of this "normal" path to a genetic legacy from infertility. In humans, there is no definitive evidence for an innate biological desire to have a child. While we have an evolutionary requirement as well as varied degrees of pride to pass on our genetic lineage, there is no assurance that genes will allow our offspring to inherit any special quality we may possess, including physical attributes, to create a "mini-me."

The human genome project identified 99% of all the genes that a human being possesses for their DNA. Through molecular testing, hundreds of human genetic mutations can be identified to provide a patient information on being a carrier of a particular disease. If the patient then conceives with a partner that carries the same genetic mutation, then their baby has a 25% chance of inheriting the full disease, some that may result in severe morbidity or mortality. Thus, pre-pregnancy genetic carrier testing can be very valuable to potentially prevent a baby from inheriting a serious disease.

The common theory to experience biological children, as opposed to non-biological, is genetics. While this is an evolutionary necessity, there is enough biological procreation to sustain the world's population to avoid any concern of a reduction in our census from those that choose third party reproduction such as egg donation and/or adoption. That is, fertile people will continue to reproduce while the one-in-eight of the population with infertility decide on how much of a physical, emotional, and financial investment they will place on building their family.

Why the emphasis on genetic testing? Because genes have an important but limited purpose in the parent-child relationship. Depending on family history, genes can place you at an inherited risk of heart disease, diabetes, and cancer, to name a few diseases. But they will not create a baby with any definitive special connection to you.

Following the successful match with our first child, I vividly remember the apprehension I experienced and the profound sense of being overwhelmed. The two questions that repeated throughout the process were, "Would I love her as if she were my "own" and would/could I ever truly bond with her?" All worries were immediately dismissed when my wife handed Mia to me – I melted and fell in love, feelings that have not abated to this day. In other words, I have learned, genes don't make a family, love does.

Third

The funk of infertility. This is how I often describe the nebulous drifting that is infertility. One becomes so accustomed to negative pregnancy tests that it becomes the norm. What's more, the funk prevents forward progression, i.e. toward IVF, egg or sperm donation, or adoption. Granted, the financial investment in treatment is prohibitive for many, particularly those who reside in states without mandated infertility insurance. The funk also contributes to the avoidance of fertility medications and treatments in favor of more natural means of procreation.

Infertility is a unique field whereby the acceptance of treatment can be as defeating as the disease. The social script is for couples to achieve pregnancy through natural conception. For many, infertility treatment is a sign of failure, i.e. an inability to have a child without assistance. Not only is this line of thinking unfair, but it also delays potential success.

I share with all my patients that my goal is not to get to know them well. The sooner the patient/couple has a successful conception, the faster they can return to their previous lifestyle, at a distance from the painful reminder of infertility.

Ten years. No one can turn back the clock. One of the greatest regrets in my life was allowing 10 years to consume our lives with infertility. Being in the field, I was so at ease with infertility treatment that enabled my wife to feel comfortable pursuing all the reproductive technology that was available. So we persevered to face incomparable disappointment and enter the abyss of despair.

Had I known my reaction to our children, I would have adopted after one to two years of infertility – or maybe sooner. However, I would, without hesitation, waited ten years for the five children that have returned life to our souls and brought more joy and fulfillment than imaginable.

Fourth

Is parenting a privilege or a right? This is an ethical debate that prompts arguments on both sides. Whichever stance a person chooses, the globally inherent approach is to love their child, irrespective of blood relation. Parents and, arguably, the community should instinctively act responsibly to maintain all children's well-being and safety.

The reality of child abuse in this country is egregious. In the US, according to data from the National Child Abuse and Neglect Data System, a child is abused or neglected every 36 seconds resulting in an average of 4 children dying per day. In 2010, "parents, acting alone or with another person, were responsible for 79.2 percent of child abuse or neglect fatalities. Almost 30 percent (29.2 percent) were perpetrated by the mother acting alone." (http://www.childabuse.com/statistics.html)

Several years ago, I performed an embryo transfer for a woman who chose to conceive by egg donation. It was a difficult decision for her following years of infertility. After I completed her procedure, she asked me that in the event she becomes pregnant, would I make sure I did not communicate with her Ob/Gyn that the baby is not hers. Her words paralyzed me on that otherwise sunny Saturday morning in Orlando. Then I asked her if we could chat a bit.

I began conveying my story of adoption and sharing my outlook that when a woman who is the intended parent holds her newborn in her arms, the baby perceives her as her mother, unequivocally and without regard to biology. The same holds true with a child born using egg donation. If the woman views the child as anything other than "hers" then she deprives the child of its primary need – unconditional love. The baby doesn't think she would be a temporary parent until its "real" parent comes along. The baby doesn't think it will be judged because it was adopted. The baby doesn't think it's a failure. So, NONE of these thoughts should EVER invade the thoughts of a parent.

If you select adoption after infertility, you are showing your acceptance of nature. This is now your chosen path of family building and the baby should NEVER be viewed as a consolation prize.

Fertility is a Gift – Not an Overstatement of Ability

The ability to reproduce is usually predetermined at birth (although infertility can be acquired) and is vital from an evolutionary standpoint. Those who view their procreative ability as prowess are misguided as to nature's circle of life. By boasting about being "Fertile Myrtle," women are claiming an accomplishment for which they had no contribution (analogous to sharing you don't have cancer) and being insensitive to those less fortunate who are struggling with infertility.

Given the myriad complicated and perilous steps in achieving a healthy newborn, one ponders how successful conception ever occurs at all. Over my long career, I have always been in awe of the complex process of human reproduction as it requires a precise and exquisitely choreographed interplay of biological mechanisms. While minor missteps are acceptable along the pathway from fertilization to embryo development to uterine implantation and ongoing pregnancy, major errors result in a failed pregnancy. Is it no wonder that the monthly pregnancy rate for a woman at her peak age of fertility is only 20%?

So, the reality is many of nature's gifts are not equally distributed, nor are they limited to otherwise exceptional recipients. If you happen to fall within the 1 in 8 who experience infertility, your options are to continue natural attempts at conception or undergo fertility treatment, both of which have the risk of resulting in child free-living while the latter can accumulate significant debt. Adoption should be proactively included in your family planning options because it is, usually, the most successful method of growing your family.

I will never know what my life would have been had we been able to experience biological children. Am I curious? Sure, but the thought does not pre-occupy me at all. What I have learned is the greatest measure of human relationship is love for the purity of loving another, wholeheartedly, without influence by biology. My prayer to all of you reading this chapter is that your journey is brief, minimally affecting the quality of your life (physically, emotionally, and financially) and your method of family building is chosen, categorically, by you.

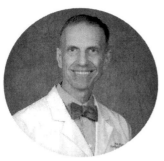

Mark Trolice, MD

Reproductive Endocrinologist and
Infertility Specialist
Author of "The Fertility Doctor's Guide
to Overcoming Infertility"

Mark Trolice, M.D. is Director of Fertility CARE: The IVF Center, an advanced reproductive technology clinic in Orlando, FL, and Professor of Ob/Gyn at the University of Central Florida College of Medicine responsible for the medical education of resident physicians and medical students. He is Board-certified in the specialty of Reproductive Endocrinology & Infertility (REI) and has been awarded the American Medical Association's "Physicians' Recognition Award" annually. In addition to his extensive publications of scientific studies and medical articles, he is a nationally recognized KOL in his field, being sought after for interviews on TV, radio, podcasts, and to speak at medical conferences. Dr. Trolice holds the unique distinction of being a fellow in the American Colleges of OB/GYN, Surgeons and Endocrinology. Physicians select him for Top Doctor in America® annually, honoring him as one among the top 5% in the U.S. His Podcast, "Fertility Health," provides the latest information in REI and, in 2020, he released, "The Fertility Doctor's Guide to Overcoming Infertility: Discovering Your Reproductive Potential and Maximizing Your Odds of Having a Baby," a book that offers unique insights from his professional and personal experiences with infertility. www.TheIVFcenter.com

An Integrative Approach to Fertility

By Dr. Melissa Wenrich

In this life, it is important to find and love ourselves. It's important to celebrate our uniqueness and the undeniable magic that flows from our souls. It's important to love the parts that may seem impossible to look upon, but when love is poured into our mind and body, we're in harmony.

Harmony is not the absence of pain and dysfunction (as we've been programmed to believe), but rather balancing all of that pain and dysfunction, along with our trauma, loss, lack of control, and our diagnosis to be used for our greatest good. Harmony is continuing to live in the present - right here, right now - amidst the autoimmune disease, PCOS, endometriosis, unexplained infertility, and loving on that very part of ourselves.

Try sitting in front of the mirror with your hand on your heart and the other on your pelvis saying aloud, you are whole. You are doing the absolute best you can at this moment. It's true, you are. It's not easy to accept. In fact, it's one of the most difficult things you'll ever do. To truly find ourselves and respect ourselves is loving and supporting and cherishing that very thing we've been told is wrong, sick, or broken.

You Are Worth It

If you're reading this, you have probably been told that something about you is broken, and because of that, I am heartbroken for you. But more so I am hopeful. I am hopeful that you can find the missing piece of information that inspires you to investigate, connect, and realize your self-worth. That missing piece that has eluded all the doctors and specialists, the predispositions of your family tree, even yourself. Whether it's a hormone imbalance, unexplained infertility, or autoimmune disease, you are so worth finding out what's missing. You are worth creating the best version of yourself; one that is strong, resilient, refreshed, peaceful, and well. You deserve to be fully seen and know without a doubt that you are only as strong as your roots and foundation. Every communication and function that is happening right now within you begins with your roots. Until we go back and take a close look at the beginning, truly dive into this process of root cause healing, we are missing out. Let's uncover your light, wellbeing, and the innate wisdom that lies within you.

Starting Slow

Starting slow may sound counterintuitive, but fertility is cumulative, collaborative, and for many very complicated, which takes time. While we are all so similar, we each have our own stories, experiences, emotional and spiritual beliefs, and genetic predispositions. All of these factors directly impact every system in our bodies and mind, influencing how we move through our day. A few of the key lifestyle elements that need to be addressed for optimal fertility include sleep, relaxation, movement, nutrition, relationships, and stress. All of these play a direct role in our brain health, which in turn affects every organ system, which if left unbalanced can lead to unwanted symptoms.

The focus of reproductive endocrinology is typically the final result or achieved pregnancy, while it routinely negates the underlying reactions in the hormone pathway and every other system that allows pregnancy to be possible. Looking into the precursors that include micronutrients, adrenals and stress response, thyroid, gut, immune system, circulation, and our musculoskeletal system are where the imbalances typically are. Yes, you may have luteal phase deficiency due to low progesterone, but why? Always ask why. This type of investigative and intuitive care and restoration takes time.

On that note, timing is key. Time may not feel like its on our side, but give yourself the time it takes to feel the best you have ever felt. We've been conditioned to think that everything happens now. Hungry? Fast food. Fever? Here's the magic pill to stop a natural and needed process. Our health is the absolute opposite of quick. When did we flip our focus to an end result instead of focusing on the fact that it takes time to bring life into the world? We would never start training for a marathon a month before the race. Yes, you might be able to do it, but at what cost? So much of our energy during TTC is on the positive test without truly assessing the health of where the egg and sperm originate. The preconception period, regardless if natural, IUI, or IVF, is six months to one year. Ideally, everyone would be able to prepare before TTC or first fertility treatment. Unfortunately, in our clinic, we are seeing new patients well into the infertility diagnosis because our current system is failing us. Don't be discouraged if this is you. Simply consider taking a break from the next transfer to focus on yourself. You don't always have to stick to a timeline, so have these discussions with your reproductive endocrinologist and advocate for what you feel is best for you.

Make the Decision to Pause

Try a route that isn't new or alternative, but foundational. According to the CDC, if you're below the age of 35 and using assisted reproductive technology, successful pregnancy rates are between 30%-45%. Financial strain aside, what can ART do when we look at mental health and stress on the body? It's in your best interest to take time for you and your partner first. The ideal preconception period is one year. During that time, necessary health issues can be explored and quality prenatal nutrients, food plans, and daily movement can be established. If In between assisted reproductive technologies, allow the proper balance to be restored before beginning the next round. The body and mind need to be well and may take time to recover from the medications. The overall components utilized in collaborative conception include a functional medicine approach, diagnostic testing and evaluation, musculoskeletal assessment including breath and blood flow patterns, and the state of your nervous system. Choosing a collaborative care model significantly shifts the chance of conception and includes a whole body, mind, and loving approach.

Make the Decision to Breathe

Breathe properly. Breathing happens unconsciously, signaled by the brain. The brain is not only keeping us alive but does so without us saying a word. We can survive (for a time) without food and water, but not without oxygen. It's the most important factor we can control regarding our health, and it's free!

The autonomic nervous system is an integral part of living, as it maintains the balance between sympathetic and parasympathetic branches of the nervous system. The sympathetic branch is our fight, flight, and freeze response, while the parasympathetic branch is our rest, digest, sex response. This is huge. We're either sitting on one or the other.

We should live within the rest/digest/sex (or parasympathetic) portion of our ANS 80% of the time. When we are here, our breath is full and diaphragmatic, our heart rate is within normal limits, digestion functioning well, and orgasm can be achieved. Circulation is flowing more within our pelvis, supplying gut and reproductive organs, and the frontal lobes of the brain are firing correctly, allowing for more critical and logical thinking, while communication within our brain and throughout our body is occurring optimally. From this state, neural pathways are rewiring and signaling appropriately.

In sympathetic mode, blood flow has shifted away from digestion, articulate brain functions, and optimized breathing, into our extremities. We're trying to outrun the bear. Or fight it. Or play dead. It's normal to feel your heartbeat speed up when something frightens you, and we can live here a portion of the time, but this cannot be homeostasis. The sympathetic nervous system allows us to survive what's in front of us. Then, when we are safe, it should shift back into parasympathetic. That shifting is adaptability and resiliency. If you find yourself unable to bring yourself back from panic, then this is an aspect of your health that needs to be addressed. Hormones require signaling from the brain. We need to be on the parasympathetic and calming side of our ANS in order to achieve optimal balance.

As mammals, we respond to stimuli differently. According to Dr. Stephen Porges' Polyvagal Theory, we can surmise that the breath - the connection of body and brain - is one of the most important aspects in achieving wellbeing. The vagus nerve, a cranial nerve that connects the brain and gut, requires proper tone. This nerve is important in digestion, how well we digest food, find calm, and breathe. Porges' work concludes that vagal nerve stimulation can be made through diaphragmatic breath, sounds, and movements. The vagus nerve plays an integral part in maintaining homeostasis with the nervous system. Recent research is emerging, which shows the impact of the vagus nerve on cardiac rhythm, bowel regulation, and inflammatory markers. We cannot outrun the very basic principle of surviving vs. thriving, no matter how many pills, supplements, and injections we consume. We cannot outsmart our nervous system. Neuroplasticity is the ability of the brain to reorganize and rewire neural pathways. Repetitive practices can increase vagal tones such as diaphragmatic breathing, singing, and gargling.

Proper breathing completely transforms the nervous system. Breath is the beginning. The majority of patients I see are not breathing fully or correctly. The diaphragm and pelvic floor work together and in unison. Try sitting comfortably with your legs crossed on your ischial tuberosity (aka your sit bones). Place your hands along your beltline and simply breathe. Don't change. Just examine. Your abdomen should expand and contract with each inhalation and exhalation. Your lower ribs, even into your back, should be moving. When you inhale your pelvic floor drops, and when you exhale it returns. Breathing not only changes the way our muscles and tendons move, but it also changes our brain function by shifting us into a calmer resting state. When this is achieved, the brain communicates within itself and the rest of the body to appropriately signal ovulation, regulate your cycle, allow for deeper sleep, and regular bowel movements.

Pelvic Floor Health

One of the key factors in reproductive health is pelvic floor circulation. If there is structural misalignment, chronically tightened muscles, or a history of previous surgeries, you more than likely aren't getting appropriate blood and lymphatic flow into your pelvic region. Some signs that tension may be present include back pain, abdominal pain, constipation, jaw or upper neck tension, trigger points in the abdominal wall, and urinary dysfunction. Chiropractic, acupuncture, fascial, and lymphatic therapies help increase blood flow and improve overall function. The research concludes that acupuncture during IUI/IVF treatments improves chances for positive pregnancy outcomes, but only if completed consistently and long term (thirteen to fifteen sessions). Once again, that's not a quick fix. Healing and improving the structure and energy of our body takes time. While ART success rates are low as stand-alone therapies, combining another form of visceral manipulation and acupuncture can double the chance of conception. In a study conducted utilizing Mercier Therapy - a soft tissue mobilization therapy - conception was achieved in over 80% of the women.

Your Health History and Testing

As a women's health practitioner, your story is the first thing we discuss in a new patient visit. After learning the timeline of your life - when you felt your best, your worst, the triggers that lead you to where you are - we make a plan to change any of the functional deficiencies or neural miscommunications you may be facing. A complete understanding of your health, social and family history, attitudes, and mental health are equally or more important than any diagnostic testing. Ideally, preconception labs should include micronutrient testing, a full panel of all hormones including adrenal, thyroid, detoxification capabilities, and genetic variants. If you have any symptoms, such as constipation/diarrhea, spotting or severe cramping with periods, irregular cycles, migraines, fatigue, inability to manage stress, or a history of synthetic birth control, these are some symptoms that may require additional testing in finding the root cause.

Basic lab testing during preconception should include: CBC, CMP, TSH, Free T4, Free T3, Reverse T3, Thyroid Peroxidase, Thyroglobulin, Prolactin, Vitamin D, Vitamin B12, Folate, Homocysteine, hs-CRP, MTHFR, Ferritin, Day 3 Estradiol, FSH, LH, SHBG, and Day 21 Progesterone. Micronutrient testing is routinely beneficial since basic pathology requires adequate nutrients and amino acids. Several studies point to improved fertility outcomes when serum Vitamin D levels are within normal functional range and that's only reviewing one of the many vital nutrients needed to thrive.

The key is understanding these labs, so find a practitioner that looks beyond the numbers. Many of these values have an enormous normal range, but if you're trending towards the lower or higher side this is a sign there is dysfunction. I don't buy into the wait and see mentality with anything in life, and especially health. We can oftentimes have symptoms of hormone dysfunction such as low libido, fatigue, hair loss, heavy periods, but lab values are classified as normal. Most physicians aren't trained in the integrative approach and the patient is told, it's in your head, you're probably anxious/depressed, and here's the pill that will hopefully help. Don't believe this methodology and realize the problem isn't you. It's the system. Step back. Find someone that's going to listen to you and what you want. Every practitioner has a purpose. The best OB/GYN's simply don't have time to help you with this so the team is critical. Not one practitioner can address all your needs. Our bodies work tirelessly to stay in harmony and find homeostasis. We can have dysfunction years before we feel the intense pain or see a number on labs shift to abnormal. If you do have anxiety, it's more than likely a result of an imbalance elsewhere.

The masking of symptoms and functionality in our healthcare system is commonplace. The fertility world is no exception. While medication is necessary in some cases, such as in thyroid disorders or insulin-dependent diabetes, many of the other uses are simply band-aids. This concept of root cause healing is very different than how most of us have been programmed. Understanding your story and getting to the root of infertility is the magic. There may be a lot of layers to uncover, many systems to explore, but you are under there. Your answer is within. Your story just needs to be heard and seen.

The hormone pathway begins with cholesterol, ending with our capability to detoxify estrogens efficiently. The adrenal, thyroid, gastrointestinal, and liver health needs proper assessments as well as a look into digestion, detoxification, micronutrients/amino acids, neurotransmitters, immune system, cell communication, the structure of organs, and musculoskeletal system. Exploring gut issues, tension headaches and lower back pain now is not only easier on the front end, but will help you feel your best during pregnancy and postpartum.

Foundational cellular health is imperative when egg and sperm quality are evaluated. Egg quality changes every 120 days and sperm around 75 days. What we consume and how well we detoxify environmental toxins contribute to their quality and our entire bodies. Toxins are one of the biggest endocrine disruptors. Transitioning from fragrances, plastics, and common household cleaners is a significant and affordable way to reduce exposure. Eating for your body is important. If you have IBS, Celiac, PCOS, blood sugar dysregulation, or other autoimmune disease finding the appropriate individualized food plan will allow you to heal more efficiently. While maintaining a healthy approach to food can be challenging if history involves disordered eating, the need to find balance and consume proper nutrients remains key. Working with a registered dietician alongside a functional medicine practitioner can ensure the plan works for you. Food is challenging, yet is the foundation of living. Society has imposed various diets for every diagnosis or goal. Be cautious. Only by knowing your full medical status can the best plan be formulated for you.

Your Team Matters

Your support team is an important relationship on your journey to parenthood. You shouldn't have to do this alone. We are not created to be alone in life. Pick your people. Feel heard by your people. The ideal team may include your obstetrician, chiropractor, acupuncturist, functional medicine practitioner, mental health practitioner, registered dietician, and reproductive endocrinologist. I know it's quite the team, but if you have been trying to conceive for longer than a year unsuccessfully, it's time to widen your net and find practitioners that specialize in fertility.

You shouldn't be the one having to beg for a new lab test you read about. There is enough stress in waiting for baby so let's shed anything unnecessary. Question everything. You have this one body and at a time emerging research is happening daily we must keep marching onward. Your team of practitioners must be open and willing to consider alternatives, communicate with one another. We need a strong village. Take time to consider who is helping you feel your best when you're with them and make your load a little bit lighter while you wait.

Love and Trust Yourself

Beginning a comprehensive and collaborative fertility approach during a difficult time can be overwhelming. Don't allow this to discourage you from moving forward. Start by allowing space to see what's best for you, build your team, and begin with foundational health. Gently open what needs to be seen and loved. Remember that our reproductive system isn't easily manipulated. We are human. We are intricate. Each and every function, thought, message relies on communication from another system to maintain harmony. Trust the innate ability of the body and that you don't need anything outside of yourself. You hold the answer. Not your doctor. Not your therapist. Only you. While we need the support of a strong team walking alongside you on this journey to empower and educate, only you hold the power to transform. Maybe begin by breathing, unravel one little piece of that balled up yarn that sits in the pit of your heart, and say to yourself, "I love you." You are worth loving. You are worth seeing your bright light and uncovering your wellbeing, and during the process of taking care of all of you, may the beautiful side effect be a healthy pregnancy and healthy child.

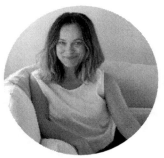

Dr. Melissa Wenrich

Chiropractic Neurologist and
Functional Medicine Practitioner
www.nashvillebrainandbody.com

Dr. Melissa Wenrich is a women's health practitioner in Nashville, TN that primarily focuses on preconception, prenatal, and postpartum care. She is a board certified chiropractic neurologist that graduated in 2005 from Logan University in St. Louis, MO. She completed her functional neurology training through the Carrick Institute and has been a diplomate with the American Board of Chiropractic Neurology since 2016. She has completed functional medicine training through the Institute of Functional Medicine and certified in acupuncture. She utilizes a functional wellness approach to support, empower, and educate women. Dr. Melissa is the founder of Nashville Brain and Body, an integrative health center in East Nashville.

The Quillet Institute

Empowering Waiting Parents To Thrive During Infertility

www.thequilletinstitute.com

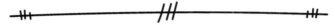

The Quillet Institute educates and empowers waiting parents through:

ONE-ON-ONE COACHING

The Quillet Institute has six, nine and twelve-week coaching packages to help you *thrive* during your season of infertility

PEACE (IN)FERTILITY PROGRAM

An 8-session online video program designed to help you live well in your wait.

PEACE (IN)FERTILITY WORKBOOK

This workbook can be used as a companion to the online program, independently, or in a group setting.

THE THRIVE SOCIETY

The Thrive Society is a space to find community, support and therapeutic tools to equip and empower its members.

THRIVE GROUPS

Thrive Groups are The Quillet Institute's version of support groups. For six weeks, women virtually join Cathie Quillet to go through the workbook Peace (In)Fertility.

THRIVE (IN)FERTILITY PODCAST

Cathie hosts the Thrive (In)Fertility podcast, interviewing others in the field of infertility and providing listeners with tools to THRIVE on their journey to parenthood.

BOOKS

Cathie Quillet is the author of, "Not Pregnant: A Companion For The Emotional Journey of Infertility" and the children's book, "No Matter What Happens," a story for when secondary infertility weaves itself into the family system.

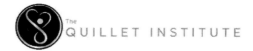